Motor Control and Learning in Childhood and Adolescence

Motor Control and Learning in Childhood and Adolescence: Interactions with Sports and Exercise

Editors

Filipe Manuel Clemente
Ana Filipa Silva

MDPI • Basel • Beijing • Wuhan • Barcelona • Belgrade • Manchester • Tokyo • Cluj • Tianjin

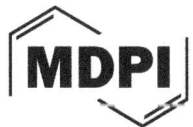

Editors
Filipe Manuel Clemente
Escola Superior de Desporto e Lazer
Instituto Politécnico de Viana do Castelo
Viana do Castelo
Portugal

Ana Filipa Silva
Escola Superior de Desporto e Lazer
Instituto Politécnico de Viana do Castelo
Viana do Casteli
Portugal

Editorial Office
MDPI
St. Alban-Anlage 66
4052 Basel, Switzerland

This is a reprint of articles from the Special Issue published online in the open access journal *Children* (ISSN 2227-9067) (available at: www.mdpi.com/journal/children/special_issues/motor_control_and_learning).

For citation purposes, cite each article independently as indicated on the article page online and as indicated below:

LastName, A.A.; LastName, B.B.; LastName, C.C. Article Title. *Journal Name* **Year**, *Volume Number*, Page Range.

ISBN 978-3-0365-3129-8 (Hbk)
ISBN 978-3-0365-3128-1 (PDF)

© 2022 by the authors. Articles in this book are Open Access and distributed under the Creative Commons Attribution (CC BY) license, which allows users to download, copy and build upon published articles, as long as the author and publisher are properly credited, which ensures maximum dissemination and a wider impact of our publications.

The book as a whole is distributed by MDPI under the terms and conditions of the Creative Commons license CC BY-NC-ND.

Contents

About the Editors vii

Preface to "Motor Control and Learning in Childhood and Adolescence: Interactions with Sports and Exercise" ix

Ghazi Rekik, Yosra Belkhir, Nourhen Mezghanni, Mohamed Jarraya, Yung-Sheng Chen and Cheng-Deng Kuo
Learning Basketball Tactical Actions from Video Modeling and Static Pictures: When Gender Matters
Reprinted from: *Children* **2021**, *8*, 1060, doi:10.3390/children8111060 1

Chia-Hui Chen, Ghazi Rekik, Yosra Belkhir, Ya-Ling Huang and Yung-Sheng Chen
Gender Differences in Attention Adaptation after an 8-Week FIFA 11+ for Kids Training Program in Elementary School Children
Reprinted from: *Children* **2021**, *8*, 822, doi:10.3390/children8090822 15

Liwa Masmoudi, Adnene Gharbi, Cyrine H'Mida, Khaled Trabelsi, Omar Boukhris and Hamdi Chtourou et al.
The Effects of Exercise Difficulty and Time-of-Day on the Perception of the Task and Soccer Performance in Child Soccer Players
Reprinted from: *Children* **2021**, *8*, 793, doi:10.3390/children8090793 27

Anja Lazić, Milovan Bratić, Stevan Stamenković, Slobodan Andrašić, Nenad Stojiljković and Nebojša Trajković
Knee Pads Do Not Affect Physical Performance in Young Female Volleyball Players
Reprinted from: *Children* **2021**, *8*, 748, doi:10.3390/children8090748 37

Lawrence Foweather, Matteo Crotti, Jonathan D. Foulkes, Mareesa V. O'Dwyer, Till Utesch and Zoe R. Knowles et al.
Foundational Movement Skills and Play Behaviors during Recess among Preschool Children: A Compositional Analysis
Reprinted from: *Children* **2021**, *8*, 543, doi:10.3390/children8070543 45

Duk-Han Ko, Yong-Chul Choi and Dong-Soo Lee
The Effect of Short-Term Wingate-Based High Intensity Interval Training on Anaerobic Power and Isokinetic Muscle Function in Adolescent Badminton Players
Reprinted from: *Children* **2021**, *8*, 458, doi:10.3390/children8060458 59

Alireza Aghababa, Georgian Badicu, Zahra Fathirezaie, Hadi Rohani, Maghsoud Nabilpour and Seyed Hojjat Zamani Sani et al.
Different Effects of the COVID-19 Pandemic on Exercise Indexes and Mood States Based on Sport Types, Exercise Dependency and Individual Characteristics
Reprinted from: *Children* **2021**, *8*, 438, doi:10.3390/children8060438 71

Hadi Nobari, Rafael Oliveira, Filipe Manuel Clemente, Jorge Pérez-Gómez, Elena Pardos-Mainer and Luca Paolo Ardigò
Somatotype, Accumulated Workload, and Fitness Parameters in Elite Youth Players: Associations with Playing Position
Reprinted from: *Children* **2021**, *8*, 375, doi:10.3390/children8050375 81

About the Editors

Filipe Manuel Clemente

Filipe Manuel Batista Clemente has been a university professor since the 2012/2013 academic year and is currently an assistant professor at Escola Superior de Desporto e Lazer de Melgaço (IPVC, Portugal). Filipe holds a Ph.D. in Sports Sciences –Sports Training from the University of Coimbra; his dissertation entitled "Towards a new approach to match analysis: understanding football players' synchronization using tactical metrics" involved observation and match analysis in soccer.

As scientific merit, Filipe has had 264 articles published and/or accepted by journals indexed with an impact factor (JCR), as well as over 105 scientific articles that have been peer-reviewed indexed in other indexes. In addition to scientific publications in journals and congresses, he is also the author of six international books and seven national books in the areas of sports training and football. He has also edited various special editions subordinate to sports training in football in journals with an impact factor and/or indexed in SCImago. Additionally, he is a frequent reviewer for impact factor journals in quartiles 1 and 2 of the JCR.

Although he started producing research in 2011, he was included in the restricted list of the world's most-cited researchers in the world (where only eight other Portuguese researchers in sports sciences appear), which was published in the journal Plos Biology in 2020. In 2021, the list was updated, with Filipe Manuel Clemente being again included in the top 2% of the world researchers, in which was positioned in the second place in six Portugueses included in the area of sports sciences. Filipe M. Clemente's SCOPUS h-index is 24 (with a total of 2605 citations), and his Google h-index is 35 (5305 citations). In a list promoted by independent website Expert Escape, he was ranked 40th of 14,875 researchers of football (soccer) in 2020 and in 19th of 15949 in 2021.

Ana Filipa Silva

Ana Filipa Silva currently works as Assistant Professor in the Polytechnic Institute of Viana do Castelo (IPVC) in Melgaço, Portugal and as a researcher in Research Centre in Sports Sciences, Health Sciences and Human Development (CIDESD, Portugal). She has a European Ph.D. in Sport Sciences –Sports Training in Faculty of Sport, University of Porto, Porto, Portugal (2017, Portugal). Among others, the main publications are within the following topics: (i) motor control, (ii) youth sports performance, (iii) decision making in sports, and (iv) cognitive performance in sports. She is currently guest associate editor for *Frontiers in Physiology*, *Frontiers in Sport,* and *Active Living and Human Movement*. She has been guest editor of many Special Issues: (i) Training and Performance in Youth Sports at International Journal Environmental Research and Public Health; (ii) In Search of Individually Optimal Movement Solutions in Sport: Learning between Stability and Flexibility at Frontiers in Physiology and Frontiers in Sport and Active Living and Human Movement; (iii) Decision-Making in Youth Sport Flexibility at Frontiers in Physiology and Frontiers in Sport and Active Living and Human Movement; and (iv) Children's Exercise Physiology, Volume II at Frontiers in Physiology and Frontiers in Sport and Active Living and Human Movement.

Preface to "Motor Control and Learning in Childhood and Adolescence: Interactions with Sports and Exercise"

The production and control of human movement is a progressive and complex process that is developed across the lifespan. New motor patterns can be learned using movement and considering the interactions with the environment. Through affordances, the human is challenged and interacts with the environment to solve problems and to improve decisions. Therefore, motor control and motor learning are two core topics that should be considered in children and young populations. Motor control is dedicated to analyzing the mastering of voluntary movement, while motor learning is more related to the process of acquiring a skill or producing a new motor task. Many types of research are produced annually on these topics. However, within the pandemic context, changes in the stimuli provided to children are the reason for concern for their development. Less free play or structured practice (e.g., sports, physical education) may have consequences for the learning and mastering of human movement. Not exclusively focusing on this situation, but opening a window to its discussion, this Special Issue "Motor Control and Learning in Childhood and Adolescence: Interactions with Sports and Exercise" aims to be a space for publishing innovative articles or systematic reviews dedicated to motor control and learning in the field of sports and exercise.

Considering that more research should be done and published about such important topics, the aim of the Special Issue "Motor Control and Learning in Childhood and Adolescence: Interactions with Sports and Exercise" was to publish high-quality original investigations, as well as narrative and systematic reviews in the field of motor control and learning in sports and exercise.

Filipe Manuel Clemente, Ana Filipa Silva
Editors

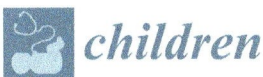

Article

Learning Basketball Tactical Actions from Video Modeling and Static Pictures: When Gender Matters

Ghazi Rekik [1,2], Yosra Belkhir [3,4], Nourhen Mezghanni [5], Mohamed Jarraya [1,6], Yung-Sheng Chen [2,7,8,*] and Cheng-Deng Kuo [2,9,10,*]

1. Research Laboratory: Education, Motricity, Sport and Health (LR19JS01), High Institute of Sport and Physical Education, Sfax University, Sfax 3000, Tunisia; ghazi.rek@gmail.com (G.R.); jarrayam@yahoo.fr (M.J.)
2. Tanyu Research Laboratory, Taipei 112, Taiwan
3. Department of Physical Education, Al-Udhailiyah Primary School for Girls, Al-Farwaniyah 085700, Kuwait; belkhir.ysr@gmail.com
4. High Institute of Sport and Physical Education, Manouba University, Manouba 2010, Tunisia
5. Department of Physical Education and Sport Science, Taif University, Taif 26571, Saudi Arabia; nsmezghanni@tu.edu.sa
6. High Institute of Sport and Physical Education, Sfax University, Sfax 3000, Tunisia
7. Department of Exercise and Health Sciences, University of Taipei, Taipei 111, Taiwan
8. Exercise and Health Promotion Association, New Taipei City 241, Taiwan
9. Department of Medical Research, Taipei Veterans General Hospital, Taipei 112, Taiwan
10. Department of Medicine, Taian Hospital, Taipei 104, Taiwan
* Correspondence: yschen@utaipei.edu.tw (Y.-S.C.); cdkuo23@gmail.com (C.-D.K.); Tel.: +886-2-2871-8288 (Y.-S.C.); +886-9-3298-1776 (C.-D.K.)

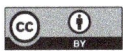

Citation: Rekik, G.; Belkhir, Y.; Mezghanni, N.; Jarraya, M.; Chen, Y.-S.; Kuo, C.-D. Learning Basketball Tactical Actions from Video Modeling and Static Pictures: When Gender Matters. *Children* 2021, *8*, 1060. https://doi.org/10.3390/children8111060

Academic Editor: Niels Wedderkopp

Received: 18 September 2021
Accepted: 15 November 2021
Published: 17 November 2021

Publisher's Note: MDPI stays neutral with regard to jurisdictional claims in published maps and institutional affiliations.

Copyright: © 2021 by the authors. Licensee MDPI, Basel, Switzerland. This article is an open access article distributed under the terms and conditions of the Creative Commons Attribution (CC BY) license (https://creativecommons.org/licenses/by/4.0/).

Abstract: Recent studies within the physical education domain have shown the superiority of dynamic visualizations over their static counterparts in learning different motor skills. However, the gender difference in learning from these two visual presentations has not yet been elucidated. Thus, this study aimed to explore the gender difference in learning basketball tactical actions from video modeling and static pictures. Eighty secondary school students (M_{age} = 15.28, SD = 0.49) were quasi-randomly (i.e., matched for gender) assigned to a dynamic condition (20 males, 20 females) and a static condition (20 males, 20 females). Immediately after watching either a static or dynamic presentation of the playing system (*learning phase*), participants were asked to rate their mental effort invested in learning, perform a game performance test, and complete the card rotations test (*test phase*). The results indicated that spatial ability (evaluated via the card rotations test) was higher in males than in female students ($p < 0.0005$). Additionally, an interaction of gender and type of visualization were identified, supporting the ability-as-compensator hypothesis: female students benefited particularly from video modeling ($p < 0.0005$, ES = 3.12), while male students did not ($p > 0.05$, ES = 0.36). These findings suggested that a consideration of a learner's gender is crucial to further boost learning of basketball tactical actions from dynamic and static visualizations.

Keywords: video modeling; static pictures; motor learning; gender difference; basketball; physical education

1. Introduction

In recent years, technology has been gaining increasing importance in different learning environments. Within the physical education (PE) domain, technology has also become an integral part of the curriculum and instruction [1]. In fact, while highly advanced and sophisticated forms of technology are generally not available during PE lessons [2], dynamic visualizations such as video modeling examples remain the more readily available didactical tools for teachers to present and explain various motor skills [3]. Video modeling involves showing the student a recording of the expert performance of a motor skill [4,5]. According to Hoogerheide et al. [6], video modeling examples seem to be very well suited for motor learning, due to their capability to deliver the information concerning how to perform a skill in an accurate way. Inspired by Bandura's social learning theory [7], a consistent body of research carried out in the PE setting has shown the effectiveness of observational learning through model-based videos. For example, it was found that video modeling examples enable inexperienced climbers to perceive and accomplish new possibilities for action and facilitate their climbing performances [8]. Moreover, a model-based video has been observed to be better than a videotaped replay of one's own performance for the acquisition and retention of the set and serve skills in volleyball [5]. Furthermore, viewing a skilled model was more effective than oral explanations for the acquisition of the shooting skill in handball [9]. In the same vein, Barzouka et al. [10] showed that observing a skilled model performing the skill of a pass in volleyball was more beneficial than oral explanations. According to Carroll and Bandura [11], observing a model would provide a perceptual blueprint of symbolic codes of the observed action. These blueprints will guide subsequent performance. In addition, Pollock and Lee [12] explained that modeling is an effective teaching method because actions which are tricky to describe verbally often can be demonstrated visually.

Despite these claims, based on the cognitive load theory [13] (a theory that considers how visual or auditory information impacts working memory and learning), Wong et al. [14] argued that videos modeling examples may not always be effective for learning, as they can become subject to transience effects. The transient information effect can be observed with videos or animations that provide a non-permanent flow of information that disappears from the computer screen [13]. Transient information requires that learners have to maintain previously presented information in WM in order to integrate it with later information [15,16]. These mental activities can overload the memory system and cause an overflow of the WM capacity [17]. The negative transient information effect provides a possible explanation as to why empirical research in the scope of cognitive load theory has suggested that replacing videos with a set of permanent/static pictures, describing the essential states of the dynamic event, may reduce the extraneous cognitive load. This instructional strategy allows learners to benefit from sufficient time to identify and process relevant information and effectively integrate it in long-term memory [18]. Moreover, viewing a series of static pictures offers the possibility to revise and compare different parts of the display as frequently as desired [19].

In this context, examining the effectiveness of video modeling vs. static pictures in learning different motor skills has raised considerable interest among sport didacticians/psychologists [20]. These scientific works dovetail nicely with findings from observational learning research. For example, Rekik et al. [21] showed that viewing skilled models performing tactical actions in basketball was more effective than viewing a series of simultaneous static pictures in terms of cognitive load, game comprehension, and attitudes (e.g., attention and enjoyment). Additionally, Rekik and his colleagues [22] recommended, whatever the complexity of the playing system, the use of video modeling examples (rather than static pictures) to teach and/or learn tactical actions in basketball. More recently, it was established that observing a skilled model performing a judo technique (through video) generated better recall-performances and guaranteed better motivation levels than different presentations of static pictures in university PE students [23,24]. The activation of the mirror neuron system has been particularly adopted by these scientists to argue the superiority of model-based videos over static visualizations (i.e., a series of photographs) in learning sport-motor knowledge/skills. This system was originally identified in primates, representing a neurophysiological circuit distributed across the pre-motor cortex that is automatically activated when someone is observing another person performing an action [25,26]. Additionally, as humans' actions are part of primary knowledge, their acquisition is very easy and requires little cognitive effort [27]. Consequently, viewing dynamic visual tools involving motor skills does not require excessive cognitive resources, because humans are biologically evolved to effectively acquire such kinds of knowledge.

The phenomenon of learning human actions through video modeling examples is referred to as "the human movement effect" [27].

The major limitation of the above-mentioned studies examining the relative effectiveness of video modeling versus static pictures in learning is that the gender of learners has not been taken into consideration. Indeed, the gender difference in learning from dynamic and static visualizations has been reported in previous educational research carried out in non-sporting domains, yielding to discrepant results [28]. On the one hand, some studies have shown that animations were especially helpful for males in geographic and problem-solving learning, indicating that while males outperformed females with the animated presentation, both genders performed similarly under static and animated presentations [29,30]. This group of scientific works supports the "ability-as-enhancer hypothesis", indicating that high spatial ability learners benefited particularly from dynamic visualizations, and low spatial ability learners did not [31,32]. Indeed, it well established that spatial ability is higher in males than females [33–37]. On the other hand, another group of studies have shown that instructional animations were particularly helpful for females in learning chemistry and physical science topics [38,39]. Similarly, it was found that there is a significant presentation–gender interaction when learning a manipulative motor skill (i.e., Lego construction task), indicating that while female students outperformed males at the completion test with video modeling, no gender differences were found with the static presentation [40]. This second group of scientific works supports the *"the ability-as-compensator hypothesis"*, indicating that low spatial ability learners (i.e., females) profited mainly from dynamic visualizations, and high spatial ability learners (i.e., males) did not [31,32,41].

While the gender difference in learning from dynamic and static visualizations was explored across a broad range of instructional domains, no explicit investigation has been conducted to examine the relationships between these two visual representations and learners' gender in learning motor skills in the PE/sport domain (i.e., motor skills requiring the whole body). We attempted to fill this knowledge gap via the present experiment, by exploring the gender difference in learning basketball tactical actions from video modeling and simultaneous static pictures in secondary school students. It was hypothesized that video modeling would be more beneficial than static pictures for learning tactical actions in basketball. It was also hypothesized that there would be a gender–instructional visualization interaction (it was an open question as to which gender would benefit most in this study due to the mixed results of previous non-sporting studies).

2. Materials and Methods
2.1. Participants

Eighty students (M_{age} = 15.28, SD = 0.49; 50% females) from a public secondary school in Tunisia completed the experimental procedure of the current study. They were selected based on sample convenience and school administrative support. The required sample size was calculated as 80 with alpha level of 0.05, the power of 0.80, and the effect size of 0.46 derived from a previous study [3]. The G*Power software (Version 3.1; Düsseldorf, Germany) was used for sample size calculations [42]. A questionnaire was used to determine the participants' demographic information and their familiarity with basketball activity and/or any other related team sports. The inclusion criteria included: (i) registered in the secondary school supporting this study; and (ii) chronological age between 14–16 years. Exclusion criteria included: (i) playing basketball or any other team ball sports in a club (this criterion was adopted to prevent transferring effects across sports [43]); and (ii) current visual impairment. Participants were informed about the study's scope, and their written informed consent to participate in this study obtained thereafter. This study was approved by the ethics committee of the Ministry of Education, Tunisia (approval code: 2173/2017). This study was undertaken in accordance with the Declaration of Helsinki and its later amendments in 2013.

2.2. Design

A 2 × 2 mixed design with factors "Condition" (video modeling vs. static pictures) and "Gender" (male vs. female) was used to investigate the hypotheses in this study. Participants were quasi-randomly (i.e., matched for gender) assigned to a dynamic condition (20 males, 20 females) and a static condition (20 males, 20 females).

2.3. Apparatus and Stimulus Information

The experiment was conducted using an HP Pavilion dv6 Entertainment PC placed at a distance of 30 cm from the participants. The stimuli (via PowerPoint software) were presented on a 32 × 20 cm screen, with a 45° viewing angle.

Participants were requested to learn how to perform different tactical actions in basketball. A structured zone attack scene was developed in collaboration with two qualified teacher/basketball coaches (with over 12 years of experience). This playing system included three players (a playmaker ①, a winger ③, and a pivot ④) who carried out a coherent tactical combination which was composed of three passes before a basket was taken through a layup. Each pass corresponded to a new step made up of multiple offensive actions achieved by the players (e.g., lateral movements, screening, and layup). Next, this game executed by three expert players (M_{age} = 21.7 years, SD = 1.26), serving as models, was filmed from a camera (using Samsung Galaxy Tab 3 SM-T211) placed above the ground from the middle of the field in an elevated position (approximately 2.5 m high). The recording position was set to film the entire field of play and all players' actions. The recorded footage was transferred onto a computer via a fire-wire connection, and then was presented into a PowerPoint page. For the static presentation version, the continuous recording was divided into four static pictures, which depicted the key steps of the playing system. Photographs were captured using FastStone Capture 6.7 software (Barcelona, Spain), and play actions were denoted by the yellow numbered arrow-symbols. A dotted arrow refers to a simple pass; a solid arrow refers to a play movement; a double solid arrow refers to a layup; and a short perpendicular line at the end of a movement line refers to a screen. These static pictures enriched with arrows (820 × 972 pixels) were displayed simultaneously in one row into a PowerPoint page (see Figure 1). The dynamic and static presentations lasted for 12 s before vanishing from the screen, and they were system paced and purely visual (i.e., without any written/spoken commentary) in order to avoid a confounding occurrence of modality, redundancy, and temporal continuity effects [44].

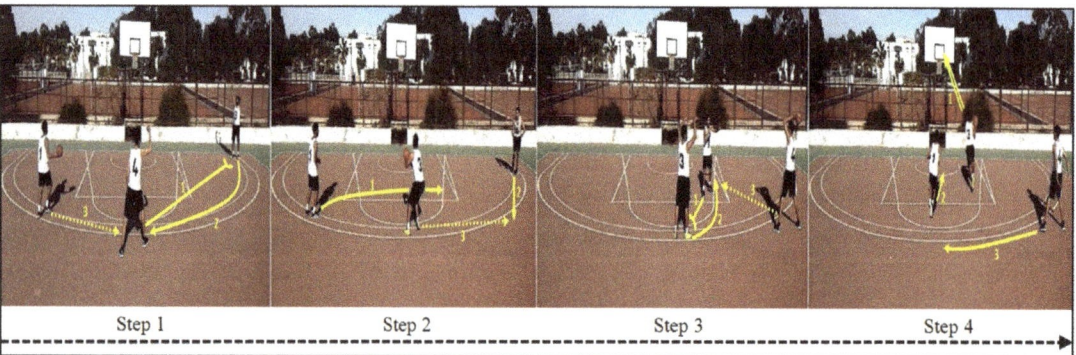

Figure 1. Sequence of four static pictures showing the four key steps of the basketball playing system.

2.4. Measurements

This study incorporated a control variable (i.e., spatial ability), and three dependent variables including, mental effort, game performance, and learning efficiency.

2.4.1. Spatial Ability

Students' spatial ability was evaluated through the card rotations test (CRT) [45]. CRT is a true–false test including two parts of 10 questions; it was developed to evaluate an individual's ability to see similarities and differences between the shapes. One point is given to each true answer, and the total scores could range from 0 to 160. Figure 2 shows one of the CRT items.

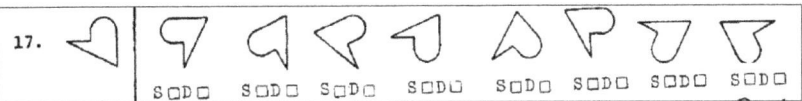

Figure 2. Example of a card rotations test item.

2.4.2. Mental Effort

A 9-point scale ranging from (1) *very, very low mental effort* to (9) *very, very high mental effort*, was used to measure the mental effort invested during the study phase. This self-rating measure is valid and reliable for estimating cognitive load [46].

2.4.3. Game Performance

A game performance task was performed in an outdoor basketball half-court, with two other male players (Mage = 16.22, SD = 1.2; semi-professional level with over 6 years of experience) who already knew the learning material. This test was conceived based on the recall–reconstruction paradigm [47]. Each tested student was instructed to reproduce as accurately as possible the tactical actions performed by a randomly chosen player from the learning material (i.e., playmaker, pivot, or winger). To guarantee the smooth running of the test, one of the semi-professional basketball players (used as teammates) was instructed to intervene by providing verbal corrective feedback each time the student performed a wrong action. A digital camera was used to record the students' game performance. Then two independent raters (qualified teacher/basketball coaches) scored the total number of correct and incorrect positions/actions. One point was awarded for each correct position/action; otherwise, participants received 0 points (see Table 1). The scores could range from 0 to 8. The inter-rater reliability was excellent and satisfactory (Cohen's κ = 0.91).

Table 1. Different steps of the basketball playing system and their related success criteria.

Steps	Criteria	Scores	
		Action	Position
1	- The pivot ④ at the level of 90° of the 3 point line on the central corridor makes a virtual pick to free the winger ③ located at the level of 0° of the 3 point line on the right side corridor	0 or 1	0 or 1
	- The winger ③ located at the level of 0° of the 3 point line on the right side corridor comes out on the pivot ④ screen and moves at the level of 90° of the 3 point line on the central corridor	0 or 1	0 or 1
	- The playmaker ① located at the level of 45° of the 3 point line on the left side corridor passes the ball to the winger ③	0 or 1	0 or 1
2	- The playmaker ① located at the level of 45° of the 3 point line on the left side corridor moves towards the "elbow" on the right side	0 or 1	0 or 1
	- The pivot ④ located at the level of 0° of the 3 point line on the right side corridor moves at the level of 45° of the 3 point line on the right side corridor	0 or 1	0 or 1
	- The winger ③ located at the level of 90° of the 3 point line on the central corridor passes the ball to the pivot ④	0 or 1	0 or 1

Table 1. Cont.

Steps		Criteria	Scores	
			Action	Position
3	-	The playmaker ① located at the "elbow" on the right side makes a virtual pick to free the winger ③ located at the level of 90° of the 3 point line on the central corridor	0 or 1	0 or 1
	-	The winger ③ located at the level of 90° of the 3 point line on the central corridor comes out on the playmaker ① screen and moves at the "elbow" on the right side	0 or 1	0 or 1
	-	The pivot ④ located at the level of 45° of the 3 point line on the right side corridor passes the ball to the winger ③	0 or 1	0 or 1
4	-	The winger ③ located at the "elbow" on the right side perform a layup	0 or 1	0 or 1
	-	The playmaker ① located at the level of 90° of the 3 point line on the central corridor moves for a rebound	0 or 1	0 or 1
	-	The pivot ④ located at the level of 45° of the 3 point line on the right side corridor moves at the level of 90° of the 3 point line on the central corridor	0 or 1	0 or 1

2.4.4. Learning Efficiency

Learning efficiency was calculated based on Kalyuga and Sweller's computational approach: Efficiency = Game performance/Mental effort [48]. These combined indicators have been seen as an optimal tool to evaluate learning from instructional visualizations [13], and have been used in previous studies assessing the effect of external visualizations on tactical learning in PE [3,4] and the sports coaching domain [49,50]. According to this computational approach, a lower mental effort investment combined with higher performance scores (and a same mental effort investment combined with higher performance scores; or vice versa) would provide evidence of a more efficient learning condition.

2.5. Procedure

The experiment was run in groups of 10 students in an outdoor basketball court. In each group, students were tested individually with the experimenter observing (±90 min), and no participant had the opportunity to observe the performance of another participant. First, each student was quasi-randomly assigned to one of the visual conditions and was instructed to memorize as precisely as possible the evolution of the scene of the play (*learning phase*). The scene of the play was shown twice resulting in a total duration of 24 s (Figure 3). Students exposed to the static pictures condition were initially informed of the functions of the arrows before watching the game situation. Immediately after watching either a static or dynamic visualization of the playing system, the student was given 30 s to indicate his/her mental effort investment level, 1 min to perform the game performance test, and 7 min to complete the card rotations test (*test phase*). The time was controlled by the experimenter using a handheld stopwatch.

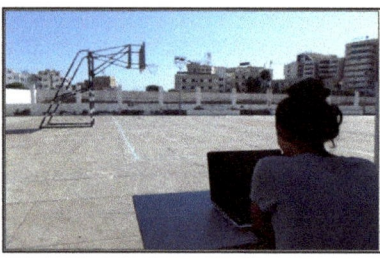

Figure 3. Learning phase.

2.6. Statistical Analyses

Statistical tests were processed using STATISTICA Software (StatSoft, Hamburg, Germany). Mean and SD (standard deviation) values were determined for each variable. After verifying that the assumptions required for parametric tests were not violated using the Shapiro–Wilk test for distribution normality, a two-way ANOVA [2 Conditions (video modeling vs. static pictures) × 2 genders (female vs. male)] with repeated measures was used to analyze the student's spatial ability, mental effort investment, game performance, and learning efficiency. When ANOVA revealed a significant difference, a post-hoc Bonferroni was applied. The qualitative magnitudes were reported as partial eta squared (n_p^2) and Cohen's mean standardized differences (ES) for post-hoc comparisons. The level of significance was set at $p < 0.05$. Following H'mida et al. [24], exact p values were reported, except when alpha level was >0.05 and/or <0.0005.

3. Results

Descriptive statistics for the control variable (i.e., spatial ability) for female and male students as a function of experimental conditions are presented in Table 2.

Table 2. Means and (standard deviations) for spatial ability, as a function of condition and gender.

	Video Modeling	Static Pictures
Male	139.4 (2.98) †	142.8 (3.97) †
Female	92.3 (4.32)	89.45 (5.03)

† Significant difference between male and female students in the same condition.

3.1. Spatial Ability

The results showed a non-significant effect of condition [$F (1.19) = 0.07$, $p > 0.05$, $n_p^2 = 0.003$], a significant effect of gender [$F (1.19) = 47.89$, $p < 0.0005$, $n_p^2 = 0.99$], and a significant interaction between these two factors [$F (1.19) = 11.90$, $p = 0.0026$, $n_p^2 = 0.38$]. Post-hoc analyses showed that the male students had significantly better spatial ability scores than the female students in the video modeling condition ($p < 0.0005$, ES = 12.69), and in the static pictures condition ($p < 0.0005$, ES = 11.77). Further analyses revealed no significant differences between the two conditions (video modeling/static pictures) for the female students ($p > 0.05$, ES = 0.60), and for the male students ($p > 0.05$, ES = 0.97). Consequently, the data analysis showed that spatial ability is higher in males than in female participants.

3.2. Game Performance

The game performance scores recorded for female and male students as a function of experimental conditions are presented in Figure 4.

The results showed a significant effect of condition [$F (1.19) = 71.55$, $p < 0.0005$, $n_p^2 = 0.79$], a significant effect of gender [$F (1.19) = 14.94$, $p = 0.0010$, $n_p^2 = 0.44$], and a significant interaction between these two factors [$F (1.19) = 15.68$, $p = 0.0008$, $n_p^2 = 0.45$]. Post-hoc analyses for the female students showed significant differences between the two conditions ($p < 0.0005$, ES = 2.30). It was found that females performed significantly better in the video modeling condition than in the static pictures condition. However, post-hoc analyses for the male students revealed no significant differences between the two conditions ($p > 0.05$, ES = 0.39). The males performed at the same level regardless of the instructional visualization (video modeling/static pictures) in which they were exposed. Further analyses showed that the female students had significantly better game performances than the male students in the video modeling condition ($p = 0.0010$, ES = 1.41). Otherwise, it was found that female and male students had similar game performances in the static pictures condition ($p > 0.05$, ES = 0.30).

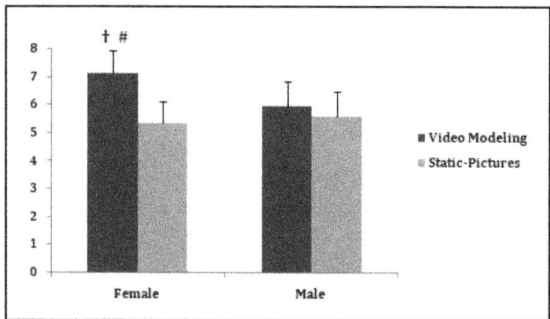

Figure 4. The game performance scores recorded for female and male students as a function of experimental conditions. # Significant difference between conditions for female students. † Significant difference between female and male students in the video modeling condition.

3.3. Mental Effort

The mental effort scores recorded for female and male students as a function of experimental conditions are presented in Figure 5.

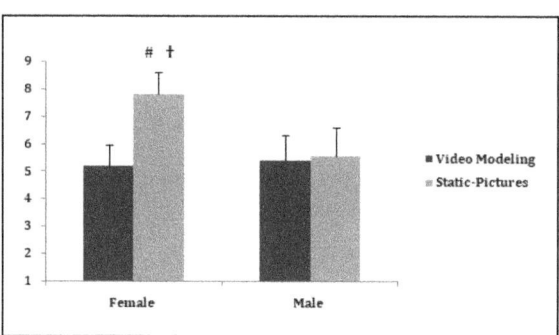

Figure 5. The mental effort scores recorded for female and male students as a function of experimental conditions. # Significant difference between conditions for female students. † Significant difference between female and male students in the static pictures condition.

The results showed a significant effect of condition [$F (1.19) = 76.12$, $p < 0.0005$, $n_p^2 = 0.80$], a significant effect of gender [$F (1.19) = 32.62$, $p < 0.0005$, $n_p^2 = 0.63$], and a significant interaction between these two factors [$F (1.19) = 61.73$, $p < 0.0005$, $n_p^2 = 0.76$]. Post-hoc analyses for the female students showed significant differences between the two conditions ($p < 0.0005$, $ES = 3.25$). It was found that females invested more mental effort in studying the static pictures condition than in the video modeling condition. However, post-hoc analyses for the male students revealed no significant differences between the two conditions ($p > 0.05$, $ES = 0.15$). The males invested the same amount of mental effort regardless of the instructional visualization (video modeling/static pictures) in which they were exposed. Further analyses showed that the female students had invested more mental effort than the male students in studying the static pictures condition ($p < 0.0005$, $ES = 2.38$). Otherwise, it was found that female and male students invested the same amount of mental effort in the video modeling condition ($p > 0.05$, $ES = 0.23$).

3.4. Learning Efficiency

The analysis showed a significant effect of condition [$F (1.19) = 80.67$, $p < 0.0005$, $n_p^2 = 0.81$], a non-significant effect of gender [$F (1.19) = 0.67$, $p > 0.05$, $n_p^2 = 0.44$], and a significant interaction between these two factors [$F (1.19) = 38.99$, $p < 0.0005$, $n_p^2 = 0.67$]. Post-hoc analyses for the female students showed significant differences between the two conditions ($p < 0.0005$, $ES = 3.12$). Therefore, for females, learning was more efficient in the video modeling condition than in the static pictures condition. However, post-hoc analyses for the male students revealed no significant differences between the two conditions ($p > 0.05$, $ES = 0.36$). The males achieved similar learning outcomes regardless of the instructional visualization (video modeling/static pictures) in which they were exposed. Further analyses showed that in the video modeling condition, learning was more efficient for the female students than for the male students ($p = 0.0050$, $ES = 1.07$). Otherwise, it was found that in the static pictures condition, learning was more efficient for the male students than for the female students ($p = 0.0006$, $ES = 1.58$). Representations based on Kalyuga and Sweller [34] of the learning efficiency measurement are illustrated in Figure 6.

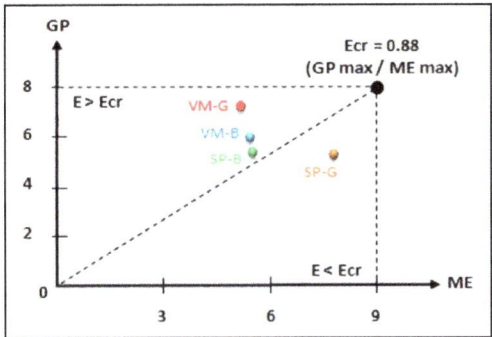

Figure 6. Learning efficiency per experimental condition for high-content complexity, based on mental effort and comprehension performance. The diagram is a representation modeled after Kalyuga and Sweller [48], where VM-G = video modeling girls, VM-B = video modeling boys, SP-G = static pictures girls, SP-B = static pictures boys, GP = game performance, ME = mental effort, E = efficiency, Ecr = critical efficiency.

4. Discussion

The study reported in this paper was designed mainly to explore how students' gender could affect tactical learning in the PE domain, when processing an offensive basketball scene from video modeling and simultaneous static pictures. To examine the relationships between these two factors (i.e., visual representations and gender), a game performance test and a self-report of mental effort scale were used.

In line with the first hypothesis, the results showed that the video modeling does not lose its effectiveness in learning basketball tactical actions (whatever the gender of the learners), despite the addition of arrow-symbols which can allow learners to improve motor learning from static pictures [24,51]. These results are in line with a consistent body of research carried out either in sports or in other instructional domains, showing the positive effects of dynamic visualizations in learning when the content to be learnt is realistic and involves procedural motor knowledge [20,21,24,52]. Consequently, the human movement effect [27] has again been supported in learning sport skills requiring the whole body, indicating that video modeling examples were found to be within the working memory constraints of the students, and were not too long and/or complex to become subject to transient effects (see Wong et al. [14] for a discussion of how the transient nature of digital videos can sometimes hinder motor learning). As mentioned in the Introduction section, the instructional/cognitive benefits of dynamic visualizations (in comparison with statics) in learning/memorizing motor skills, were principally due to the activation of the mirror neuron system [25,26].

An additional crucial finding of the current study was the significant interaction between gender and visualization formats, indicating that while females performed better with the video modeling than with static pictures (i.e., they achieved higher game performances with less mental effort investment), males did not gain particular benefits from dynamic presentation (i.e., they achieved the same game performances with the same amount of mental effort investment). These results are consistent with previous research indicating that females profited particularly from dynamic visualizations (and males did not) in learning descriptive knowledge [38,39]. More importantly, our results are in accordance with Wong et al. [40] showing that females outperformed males with the video modeling, and that no gender differences were found with the static pictures, in learning a manipulative motor skill (i.e., Lego construction task). To explain these results, it is indispensable to refer to the student's individual spatial ability that was evaluated as a control variable in our study through the CRT developed by Ekstrom et al. [45]. Indeed, it is interesting to note that males achieved better scores than females in the CRT, confirming the results of previous works indicating that spatial ability is higher in males than in females [33–36]. Consequently, our findings could support the *"ability-as-compensator hypothesis"*, indicating that low spatial ability learners (i.e., females) profited mainly from dynamic visualizations, and high spatial ability learners (i.e., males) did not [31,32,41]. Following this hypothesis, dynamic formats can further boost the learning of students with low spatial ability by offering an explicit and continuous representation of the spatio-temporal elements of the system, and thereby, avoiding the process of mental inference from static presentation formats. Yet, dynamic and static visualizations can have similar effects on learning among students with high spatial ability as they are more cognitively prepared to generate an adequate mental representation of the learning content whatever the presentation format [32]. Another plausible explanation for the superiority of female over male students in learning from video modeling could be related to the anatomical differences in the mirror neuron system. It is well known that the female brain has a higher proportion (compared to male brain) of gray matter in the prefrontal cortex [53,54], which play a crucial role in human attention [55]. As attention is the first necessary condition in any form of observing and modeling behavior [7], it is logical to have found that females achieved higher learning outcomes than males when processing a basketball playing system from video modeling examples. However, it should be cautioned that this study did not include any anatomical brain data, leaving it partially speculative. Further research is needed to explore this issue by using objective measures (e.g., [56]).

Some limitations should be mentioned as is the case for all experimental research. First, in the current study we focused solely on spatial ability as potential gender cognitive variables that can influence the learning from dynamic vs. static visualizations due to its large documented impact. However, it was established that there are both biological and social differences in the ways that males and females process external stimuli [57]. Second, the participants' age may be a limiting factor for the generalization of our results' interpretation. Additional research on this topic should perhaps explore this pattern of results with children or older participants (e.g., university PE students). Third, the current investigation was based on the conventional learning-and-recall experimental procedure [3]. In other words, participants were asked to perform the recall-performance test immediately after they had just watched one of the two visual supports. It would be worthwhile in future studies to examine findings of this study in a real-world setting (i.e., during regular PE lessons). Lastly, all participants undertook the experimental procedure at the same time of the day (i.e., in the morning). Further studies are required to investigate the effects of the time of the day and instructional visualizations (i.e., static vs. dynamic) in learning about basketball tactical skills, because it was established that cognitive abilities such as reaction time, attention, and executive functions depend heavily on the time of the day [58].

5. Conclusions

The current study extends the existing research examining the relationships between instructional visualizations and gender, indicating a significant interaction between these two factors in learning sport-specific motor skills (basketball tactical actions). For female secondary school students, learning was more efficient with video modeling than with static pictures. However, male secondary school students achieved similar learning performances with both types of instructional visualizations. In summary, this study suggests that a consideration of learners' gender is crucial to further boost learning of basketball tactical actions from dynamic and static visualizations in adolescent students.

Author Contributions: Conceptualization, G.R.; methodology, G.R.; software, G.R.; investigation, G.R. and Y.B.; statistical analysis, Y.B.; data interpretation, G.R.; writing—original draft preparation, G.R. and Y.B; writing-review and editing, G.R., N.M., Y.-S.C. and C.-D.K.; supervision, M.J., Y.-S.C. and C.-D.K.; project administration, G.R. All authors have read and agreed to the published version of the manuscript.

Funding: This research was funded by Taipei Veterans General Hospital, grant number V95S1-013.

Institutional Review Board Statement: The study was conducted according to the guidelines of the Declaration of Helsinki, and approved by the ethics committee of the Ministry of Education, Tunisia (approval code: 2173/2017; Date: 9 October 2017).

Informed Consent Statement: Informed consent was obtained from all subjects involved in the study.

Data Availability Statement: The data are available upon request to the corresponding author's email.

Acknowledgments: We would like to thank the students involved for their efforts, commitment, and enthusiasm throughout the study. We would also like to thank the PE teacher "Fahmi Ellouze" for his cooperation and technical assistance.

Conflicts of Interest: The authors declare no conflict of interest.

References

1. Papastergiou, M. Enhancing physical education and sport science students' self-efficacy and attitudes regarding information and communication technologies through a computer literacy course. *Comput. Educ.* **2010**, *54*, 298–308. [CrossRef]
2. Palao, J.M.; Hastie, P.A.; Cruz, P.G.; Ortega, E. The impact of video technology on student performance in physical education. *Technol. Pedagogy Educ.* **2015**, *24*, 51–63. [CrossRef]
3. Rekik, G.; Belkhir, Y.; Jarraya, M. Searching to improve learning from complex animated basketball scenes: When decreasing the presentation speed is more efficient than using segmentation. *Technol. Pedagogy Educ.* **2021**, *30*, 1–15. [CrossRef]
4. Jarraya, M.; Rekik, G.; Belkhir, Y.; Chtourou, H.; Nikolaidis, P.T.; Rosemann, T.; Knechtle, B. Which presentation speed is better for learning basketball tactical actions through video modeling examples? The influence of content complexity. *Front. Psychol.* **2019**, *10*, 2356. [CrossRef]
5. Zetou, E.; Tzetzis, G.; Vernadakis, N.; Kioumourtzoglou, E. Modeling in learning two volleyball skills. *Percept. Mot. Ski.* **2002**, *94*, 1131–1142. [CrossRef] [PubMed]
6. Hoogerheide, V.; van Wermeskerken, M.; Loyens, S.M.; van Gog, T. Learning from video modeling examples: Content kept equal, adults are more effective models than peers. *Learn. Instr.* **2016**, *44*, 22–30. [CrossRef]
7. Bandura, A. Self-efficacy: Toward a unifying theory of behavioral change. *Psychol. Rev.* **1977**, *84*, 191–215. [CrossRef] [PubMed]
8. Boschker, M.S.; Bakker, F.C.; Michaels, C.F. Memory for the functional characteristics of climbing walls: Perceiving affordances. *J. Mot. Behav.* **2002**, *34*, 25–36. [CrossRef]
9. Nahid, S.; Zahra, N.R.; Elham, A. Effects of video modeling on skill acquisition in learning the handball shoot. *Eur. J. Exp. Biol.* **2013**, *3*, 214–218.
10. Barzouka, K.; Sotiropoulos, K.; Kioumourtzoglou, E. The effect of feedback through an expert model observation on performance and learning the pass skill in volleyball and motivation. *J. Phys. Educ. Sport* **2015**, *15*, 3.
11. Carroll, W.R.; Bandura, A. Representational guidance of action production in observational learning: A causal analysis. *J. Mot. Behav.* **1990**, *22*, 85–97. [CrossRef]
12. Pollock, B.J.; Lee, T.D. Effects of the model's skill level on observational motor learning. *Res. Q. Exerc. Sport* **1992**, *63*, 25–29. [CrossRef]
13. Sweller, J.; Van Merrienboer, J.J.; Paas, F.G. Cognitive architecture and instructional design. *Educ. Psychol. Rev.* **1998**, *10*, 251–296. [CrossRef]
14. Wong, A.; Leahy, W.; Marcus, N.; Sweller, J. Cognitive load theory, the transient information effect and e-learning. *Learn. Instr.* **2012**, *22*, 449–457. [CrossRef]
15. Ayres, P.; Paas, F. Making instructional animations more effective: A cognitive load approach. *Appl. Cogn. Psychol.* **2007**, *21*, 695–700. [CrossRef]
16. Moreno, R.; Mayer, R. Interactive multimodal learning environments. *Educ. Psychol. Rev.* **2007**, *19*, 309–326. [CrossRef]
17. Baddeley, A. Working memory: Looking back and looking forward. *Nat. Rev. Neurosci.* **2003**, *4*, 829–839. [CrossRef] [PubMed]

18. Mayer, R.E.; DeLeeuw, K.E.; Ayres, P. Creating retroactive and proactive interference in multimedia learning. *Appl. Cogn. Psychol.* **2007**, *21*, 795–809. [CrossRef]
19. Carpenter, P.A.; Shah, P. A model of the perceptual and conceptual processes in graph comprehension. *J. Exp. Psychol. Appl.* **1998**, *4*, 75–100. [CrossRef]
20. Rekik, G.; Belkhir, Y.; Jarraya, M.; Bouzid, M.A.; Chen, Y.S.; Kuo, C.D. Uncovering the Role of Different Instructional Designs When Learning Tactical Scenes of Play through Dynamic Visualizations: A Systematic Review. *Int. J. Environ. Res. Public Health* **2021**, *18*, 256. [CrossRef]
21. Rekik, G.; Khacharem, A.; Belkhir, Y.; Bali, N.; Jarraya, M. The instructional benefits of dynamic visualizations in the acquisition of basketball tactical actions. *J. Comput. Assist. Learn.* **2019**, *35*, 74–81. [CrossRef]
22. Rekik, G.; Khacharem, A.; Belkhir, Y.; Bali, N.; Jarraya, M. The effect of visualization format and content complexity on acquisition of tactical actions in basketball. *Learn. Motiv.* **2019**, *65*, 10–19. [CrossRef]
23. H'mida, C.; Degrenne, O.; Souissi, N.; Rekik, G.; Trabelsi, K.; Jarraya, M.; Bragazzi, N.L.; Khacharem, A. Learning a Motor Skill from Video and Static Pictures in Physical Education Students—Effects on Technical Performances, Motivation and Cognitive Load. *Int. J. Environ. Res. Public Health* **2020**, *17*, 9067. [CrossRef] [PubMed]
24. H'mida, C.; Kalyuga, S.; Souissi, N.; Rekik, G.; Jarraya, M.; Khacharem, A. Is the human movement effect stable over time? The effects of presentation format on acquisition and retention of a motor skill. *J. Comput. Assist. Learn.* **2021**. [CrossRef]
25. Rizzolatti, G.; Craighero, L. The mirror-neuron system. *Annu. Rev. Neurosci.* **2004**, *27*, 169–192. [CrossRef]
26. Van-Gog, T.; Paas, F.; Marcus, N.; Ayres, P.; Sweller, J. The mirror neuron system and observational learning: Implications for the effectiveness of dynamic visualizations. *Educ. Psychol. Rev.* **2009**, *21*, 21–30. [CrossRef]
27. Paas, F.; Sweller, J. An evolutionary upgrade of cognitive load theory: Using the human motor system and collaboration to support the learning of complex cognitive tasks. *Educ. Psychol. Rev.* **2012**, *24*, 27–45. [CrossRef]
28. Castro-Alonso, J.C.; Wong, M.; Adesope, O.O.; Ayres, P.; Paas, F. Gender imbalance in instructional dynamic versus static visualizations: A meta-analysis. *Educ. Psychol. Rev.* **2019**, *31*, 361–387. [CrossRef]
29. Griffin, A.L.; MacEachren, A.M.; Hardisty, F.; Steiner, E.; Li, B. A comparison of animated maps with static small-multiple maps for visually identifying space-time clusters. *Ann. Am. Assoc. Geogr.* **2006**, *96*, 740–753. [CrossRef]
30. Lin, C.F.; Hung, Y.H.; Chang, R.I.; Hung, S.H. Developing a problem-solving learning system to assess the effects of different materials on learning performance and attitudes. *Comput. Educ.* **2014**, *77*, 50–66. [CrossRef]
31. Mayer, R.E.; Sims, V.K. For whom is a picture worth a thousand words? Extensions of a dual-coding theory of multimedia learning. *J. Educ. Psychol.* **1994**, *86*, 389–401. [CrossRef]
32. Höffler, T.N. Spatial ability: Its influence on learning with visualizations—a meta-analytic review. *Educ. Psychol. Rev.* **2010**, *22*, 245–269. [CrossRef]
33. Linn, M.C.; Petersen, A.C. Emergence and characterization of sex differences in spatial ability: A meta-analysis. *Child Dev.* **1985**, *56*, 1479–1498. [CrossRef] [PubMed]
34. Feng, J.; Spence, I.; Pratt, J. Playing an action video game reduces gender differences in spatial cognition. *Psychol. Sci.* **2007**, *18*, 850–855. [CrossRef] [PubMed]
35. Campbell, S.M.; Collaer, M.L. Stereotype threat and gender differences in performance on a novel visuospatial task. *Psychol. Women. Q.* **2009**, *33*, 437–444. [CrossRef]
36. Uttal, D.H.; Meadow, N.G.; Tipton, E.; Hand, L.L.; Alden, A.R.; Warren, C.; Newcombe, N.S. The Malleability of spatial skills: A Meta-analysis of training studies. *Psychol. Bull.* **2013**, *139*, 352–402. [CrossRef]
37. Voyer, D.; Hou, J. Type of items and the magnitude of gender differences on the Mental Rotations Test. *Can. J. Exp. Psychol.* **2006**, *60*, 91–100. [CrossRef]
38. Yezierski, E.J.; Birk, J.P. Misconceptions about the particulate nature of matter: Using animations to close the gender gap. *J. Chem. Educ.* **2006**, *83*, 954–960. [CrossRef]
39. Sánchez, C.A.; Wiley, J. Sex differences in science learning: Closing the gap through animations. *Learn. Individ. Differ.* **2010**, *20*, 271–275. [CrossRef]
40. Wong, M.; Castro-Alonso, J.C.; Ayres, P.; Paas, F. Gender effects when learning manipulative tasks from instructional animations and static presentations. *J. Educ. Techno. Soc.* **2015**, *18*, 37–52.
41. Höffler, T.N.; Leutner, D. The role of spatial ability in learning from instructional animations–Evidence for an ability-as-compensator hypothesis. *Comput. Hum. Behav.* **2011**, *27*, 209–216. [CrossRef]
42. Faul, F.; Erdfelder, E.; Buchner, A.; Lang, A.G. Statistical power analyses using G* Power 3.1: Tests for correlation and regression analyses. *Behav. Res. Methods* **2009**, *41*, 1149–1160. [CrossRef] [PubMed]
43. Smeeton, N.J.; Ward, P.; Williams, A.M. Do pattern recognition skills transfer across sports? A preliminary analysis. *J. Sports Sci.* **2004**, *22*, 205–213. [CrossRef] [PubMed]
44. Kalyuga, S. Relative effectiveness of animated and static diagrams: An effect of learner prior knowledge. *Comput. Hum. Behav.* **2008**, *24*, 852–861. [CrossRef]
45. Ekstrom, R.B.; Dermen, D.; Harman, H.H. *Manual for Kit of Factor-Referenced Cognitive Tests*, 1st ed.; Educational Testing Service: Princeton, NJ, USA, 1976; pp. 147–149.
46. Paas, F. Training strategies for attaining transfer of problem-solving skill in statistics: A cognitive-load approach. *J. Educ. Psychol.* **1992**, *84*, 429–434. [CrossRef]

47. Chase, W.G.; Simon, H.A. Perception in chess. *Cogn. Psychol.* **1973**, *4*, 55–81. [CrossRef]
48. Kalyuga, S.; Sweller, J. Rapid dynamic assessment of expertise to improve the efficiency of adaptive e-learning. *Educ. Technol. Res. Dev.* **2005**, *53*, 83–93. [CrossRef]
49. Rekik, G.; Belkhir, Y.; Mnif, M.; Masmoudi, L.; Jarraya, M. Decreasing the Presentation Speed of Animated Soccer Scenes Does Not Always Lead to Better Learning Outcomes in Young Players. *Int. J. Hum. Comput. Int.* **2020**, *36*, 717–724. [CrossRef]
50. Rekik, G.; Belkhir, Y.; Jarraya, M. Improving Soccer Knowledge from Computerized Game Diagrams: Benefits of Sequential Instructional Arrows. *Percept. Mot. Ski.* **2021**, *128*, 912–931. [CrossRef]
51. Garland, T.B.; Sanchez, C.A. Rotational perspective and learning procedural tasks from dynamic media. *Comput. Educ.* **2013**, *69*, 31–37. [CrossRef]
52. Boucheix, J.M.; Forestier, C. Reducing the transience effect of animations does not (always) lead to better performance in children learning a complex hand procedure. *Comput. Hum. Behav.* **2017**, *69*, 358–370. [CrossRef]
53. Gur, R.C.; Turetsky, B.I.; Matsui, M.; Yan, M.; Bilker, W.; Hughett, P.; Gur, R.E. Sex differences in brain gray and white matter in healthy young adults: Correlations with cognitive performance. *J. Neurosci.* **1999**, *19*, 4065–4072. [CrossRef]
54. Solianik, R.; Brazaitis, M.; Skurvydas, A. Sex-related differences in attention and memory. *Medicina* **2016**, *52*, 372–377. [CrossRef]
55. Kanai, R.; Rees, G. The structural basis of inter-individual differences in human behaviour and cognition. *Nat. Rev. Neurosci.* **2011**, *12*, 231–242. [CrossRef] [PubMed]
56. Hadjikhani, N.; Joseph, R.M.; Snyder, J.; Tager-Flusberg, H. Anatomical differences in the mirror neuron system and social cognition network in autism. *Cereb. Cortex.* **2006**, *16*, 1276–1282. [CrossRef] [PubMed]
57. Bevilacqua. Commentary: Should gender differences be included in the evolutionary upgrade to cognitive load theory? *Educ. Psychol. Rev.* **2017**, *29*, 189–194. [CrossRef]
58. Jarraya, S.; Jarraya, M. The effects of music and the time-of-day on cognitive abilities of tennis player. *Int. J. Sport. Exerc. Psychol.* **2019**, *17*, 185–196. [CrossRef]

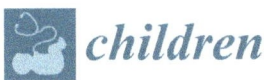

Article

Gender Differences in Attention Adaptation after an 8-Week FIFA 11⁺ for Kids Training Program in Elementary School Children

Chia-Hui Chen [1], Ghazi Rekik [2,3], Yosra Belkhir [2,4,5], Ya-Ling Huang [6] and Yung-Sheng Chen [7,8,*]

1. Sporting Education Office, National Taiwan University of Science and Technology, Taipei 10607, Taiwan; monkey0209@gmail.com
2. Research Laboratory: Education, Motricity, Sport and Health, LR19JS01, Sfax University, Sfax 3000, Tunisia; ghazi.rek@gmail.com (G.R.); belkhir.ysr@gmail.com (Y.B.)
3. Tanyu Research Laboratory, Taipei 11266, Taiwan
4. Al-Udhailiyah Primary School for Girls, Al-Farwaniyah 085700, Kuwait
5. High Institute of Sport and Physical Education, Manouba University, Manouba 2010, Tunisia
6. Sporting Education Office, Chang Gung University of Science and Technology, Taoyuan 33303, Taiwan; ylhuang@mail.cgust.edu.tw
7. Department of Exercise and Health Sciences, University of Taipei, Taipei 111036, Taiwan
8. Exercise and Health Promotion Association, New Taipei City 24156, Taiwan
* Correspondence: yschen@utaipei.edu.tw; Tel.: +886-2-2871-8288 (ext. 6405)

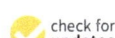

Citation: Chen, C.-H.; Rekik, G.; Belkhir, Y.; Huang, Y.-L.; Chen, Y.-S. Gender Differences in Attention Adaptation after an 8-Week FIFA 11⁺ for Kids Training Program in Elementary School Children. *Children* **2021**, *8*, 822. https://doi.org/10.3390/children8090822

Academic Editor: Zoe Knowles

Received: 14 July 2021
Accepted: 15 September 2021
Published: 18 September 2021

Publisher's Note: MDPI stays neutral with regard to jurisdictional claims in published maps and institutional affiliations.

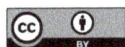

Copyright: © 2021 by the authors. Licensee MDPI, Basel, Switzerland. This article is an open access article distributed under the terms and conditions of the Creative Commons Attribution (CC BY) license (https://creativecommons.org/licenses/by/4.0/).

Abstract: School-based exercise intervention is recognized as an optimal tool for enhancing attentional performance in healthy school children. However, gender differences in the training adaptation regarding attentional capacities have not been elucidated clearly in the current literature. This study aimed to investigate the effects of an 8-week Fédération Internationale de Football Association (FIFA) 11⁺ for Kids training program on attentional performance in schoolboys and girls. Based on a quasi-experimental design, fifty-two children registered in year five of elementary school were assigned into the following groups: training boys ($n = 13$), training girls ($n = 13$), control boys ($n = 13$) and control girls ($n = 13$). The training groups undertook an 8-week FIFA 11⁺ Kids intervention with a training frequency of five times per week, whereas the control groups were deprived of any exercise during the study period. All the participants maintained their regular physical activity and weekly physical education (PE) lessons (two 50-min lessons per week of school curriculum) during the training period. The Chinese version of the Attention Scale for Elementary School Children (ASESC) test was used for attentional assessment at the baseline and one week after the interventional period. The Kruskal–Wallis H test was used for between-group comparison, whereas the Wilcoxon signed-rank test was used for within-group comparison. Significant differences in total scale, focused attention, selective attention, and alternating attention were found in group comparisons ($p < 0.001$). Furthermore, the training children significantly increased their values in relation to total scale, focused attention, sustained attention, and selective attention ($p < 0.05$). Only training girls significantly improved their divided attention after the training period ($p < 0.001$, MD = −0.77, ES = −0.12). In conclusion, the FIFA 11⁺ for Kids is an effective school-based exercise intervention for attentional improvement in school children. The schoolgirls demonstrated a positive outcome regarding divided attention after the interventional period.

Keywords: school-based exercise; pediatric health; concentration; gender difference; exercise intervention

1. Introduction

A fundamental aspect of school education is related to the attention and learning efficiency of students. Two questions that are always uppermost in all educators' and parents' minds are as follows: "Does this child have attention problems? How do I improve the attention span for children learning at school?" In the 1970s, Posner [1] stated that an attentional process involves multiple cognitive functions in the central nervous system. Later, a framework proposed by Posner and his colleagues [2] outlined a holistic representation of attention networks including alerting, orienting, and executive control aspects. Neurophysiological studies, particularly in neuroanatomic, neuroimaging and neurobiological evidence support the role of cerebral functions associated with attentional control [3]. For example, biogenetic studies have reported that biological factors, such as dopamine D4 receptor (DRD4), dopamine transporter (DAT1), catecholamine-O-methyl transferase (COMT), and monoamine oxidase (MAOA), are related to psychological behavior and attention functions [4,5].

Attentional modulation and plasticity in the human brain are evidenced by attentional training interventions and a proper learning environment in the early stages of growth [6,7]. During development, preadolescent boys display different characteristics regarding attentional performance in comparison to preadolescent girls; these differences are due to physiological, psychological, and social aspects. For example, Clarke et al. [8] reported that schoolboys showed fewer theta electroencephalography (EEG) brainwaves and more alpha EEG brainwaves than schoolgirls, indicating gender differences in brain function during childhood. Additionally, gender differences in attentional control have been found in children with attention deficit hyperactivity disorder (ADHD) (i.e., girls had lower Conners ADHD rating scales) [9]. It is well documented that daily physical activities and exercise interventions are strongly related to attentional performance in school-aged children [10–13]. In acute exercise intervention, a 12-min continuous running exercise can immediately improve selective attention in children [14]. Additionally, an acute bout of 20-min treadmill walking at a moderate intensity of 60% maximal heart rate results in functional improvement in attentional tasks in 10-year-old children [15]. The modulation of exercise-induced neurotransmitters in the cerebrum (such as adrenaline, dopamine, and brain-derived neurotrophic factors) is considered a primary mechanism to alter post-exercise attentional performance [16,17]. In terms of the chronic effects of exercise intervention, a longitudinal study reported that developing executive function skills before and during school age was strongly associated with elementary school mathematics performance, indicating the important role of attention and motor performance in the early development of school children [18]. Moreover, school-based exercise interventions can contribute to beneficial outcomes regarding attention control and academic performance in school-aged children [19]. Superior cognitive improvements and higher levels of physical engagement were also identified in school children who undertook a 6-week team game in comparison to those who undertook 6 weeks of aerobic exercise [20]. The cognitive benefits of chronic exercise interventions in children have been suggested as being a result of exercise-induced adaptation in cognitive–motor interactions of cerebral regions, such as the prefrontal cortex, motor cortex, and basal ganglia [21]. This assumption has been evidenced by an increase in spatial working memory after an 8-week gymnastics training program in school children [22].

The Fédération Internationale de Football Association (FIFA) 11$^+$ for Kids is a structured training program with the aim of improving neuromuscular functions in preadolescent children [23,24]. Recent studies have reported on chronological adaptation in enhancing skill-related physical fitness components of youth football players [25–27]. For example, Rössler et al. [25] found that footballers aged 7–12 significantly improved their Y-balance capacity, jumping ability, agility, and dribbling ability after a 10-week FIFA 11$^+$ for Kids program. However, the optimal benefits regarding the physiological adaptation of the FIFA 11$^+$ for Kids were only reported in sports trained youth players. Recently, our laboratory [28] conducted an intensive 8-week FIFA 11$^+$ for Kids training program in elementary school children. Our findings reported the positive benefits of physical fitness (e.g., sit-and-reach, broad jump, sit-up, and 800 m run) and attentional capacity. This finding implies that structure-based exercise interventions can positively improve attentional performance in school children.

To the best of our knowledge, information regarding the influence of gender differences in exercise training adaptations on attentional control has not yet been elucidated in the literature, particularly in relation to school children. Most importantly, we seek to identify which area of attentional performance can help schoolteachers deliver appropriate course curricula to approach the demands of individual children. Therefore, the purpose of this study was to compare gender differences in attentional adaptation after an 8-week FIFA 11+ for Kids training intervention in elementary school children. The secondary purpose of this study was to identify what attentional capacity could be adaptable to the exercise intervention. It was first hypothesized that the 8-week FIFA 11+ for Kids would enhance attentional capacities in training children. The second hypothesis was that training girls would be superior in terms of training adaptation in all attentional assessments, compared to training boys and control children.

2. Materials and Methods

2.1. Participants

Fifty-two healthy children from a public elementary school voluntarily participated in this study (Sanchong district, New Taipei City, Taiwan). Based on a quasi-experimental design, thirteen children of the same gender were assigned into the FIFA 11+ for Kids Boys (training boys) group, the FIFA 11+ for Kids girls (training girls) group, control boys group, or control girls group (see Figure 1).

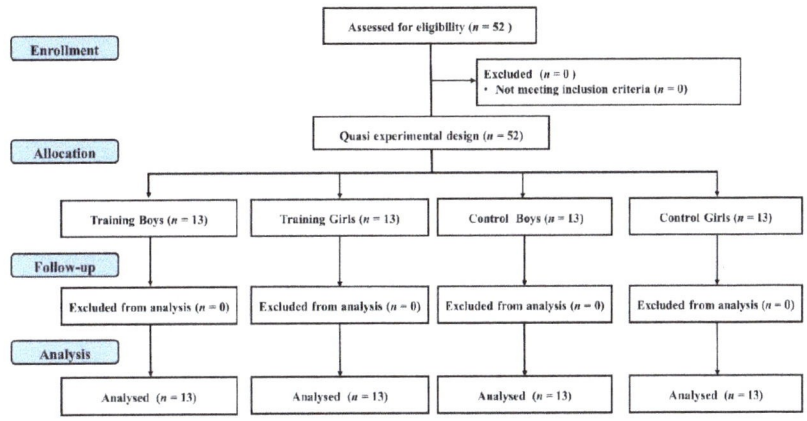

Figure 1. Experimental flow diagram of the study.

The inclusion criteria were as follows: (1) registered in the fifth year of elementary school; and (2) chronological age between 10–12. Exclusion criteria included the following: (1) current neurological or cardiovascular diseases; (2) psychological disorders; (3) taking medicine that affects psychometric status (e.g., benzodiazepines, anticonvulsants, antidepressants).

Prior to the experiment, all children and their parents and schoolteachers were informed of the scope of the study and the experimental procedure. All children were screened and there were no contraindications to participation. All children and parents signed informed consent forms. Subsequently, the children were familiarized with the experimental tests. This study was approved by the Human Research Ethics Committee of University of Taipei (UT-IRB-2020-003). This study was undertaken in accordance with the Declaration of Helsinki and its later amendments in 2013.

2.2. Experimental Procedure

The study was conducted during the spring semester of the school year. Based on the school curriculum and teaching schedule, one class of 26 children with an equal number of boys and girls was allocated to the training groups while another 13 boys and 13 girls from another class were assigned to the control groups. During the baseline stage, the participants undertook anthropometrics measurements for height (Seca 213; seca GmbH and Co. KG, Hamburg, Germany) and body weight (Xyfwt382; TECO, Taiwan) in the school health center. Afterwards, the participants performed the Chinese version of the Attention Scale for Elementary School Children (ASESC) test for attentional assessments in their classrooms. The participants were given hard copies of ASESC testing sheets and a pencil to complete the attentional assessment. The duration of the ASESC test was around 50 min in total (including resting intervals and ten tasks). The following week, the training groups began an 8-week FIFA 11+ kid intervention with a training frequency of five times per week. Conversely, participants in the control groups were deprived of any exercise intervention during the study period. All participants were told to maintain their regular physical activity and physical education (PE) lessons (two 50-minutee lessons per week of school curriculum) during the training period. A post-training ASESC test was conducted a week after the training period, following the same testing procedures as the baseline measurement. The participants were asked to refrain from strenuous exercises 24 h before the baseline and post-training assessments. A research assistant was blinded to conduct the ASESC tests in this study. One research fellow evaluated the score of attentional assessment in accordance with the ASESC test guidelines. Figure 1 shows the experimental flow of the study.

2.3. Training Intervention

The FIFA 11+ for Kids exercise program was used as a training intervention in this study. The program consisted of seven types of motor coordination exercises (running, skating jumps, single-leg stance, push-ups, single-leg jumps, spiderman, and sideways roll) with five variations (from basic to advance) [23]. Overall, a total of 35 exercises were included in the exercise program. The details of the FIFA 11+ for Kids intervention, as used in a school exercise program, are described in our recent publication [28].

During the training period, each training session (lasting 40-min) was conducted by a physical education teacher and a research assistant, both of whom were familiar with the FIFA 11+ for Kids program. The training boys and girls were instructed with appropriate movement operation and performance skills during training sessions. All training sessions started with a roll call at 8:00 a.m. on school days. All training boys and girls fully attended the training sessions during the training period.

2.4. Attentional Assessment

The Chinese version of the ASESC test developed by Lin and Chou [29] was used as an attentional assessment tool in this study. This scale is a reliable tool for a multi-dimensional attention test based on the "Clinical Attention Model" proposed by Sohlberg and Mateer [30,31]. The ASESC test consists of ten variants of attentional tasks (from item 1 to item 10) and is divided into (1) focused attention (item 1 and 2, 1 min for each test); (2) sustained attention (item 3 and 4, 5 min for each test); (3) selective attention (item 5 and 6, 1 min for each test); (4) alternating attention (item 7 and 8, 1 min for each test); and (5) divided attention (item 9 and 10, 2.5 min for each test).

Focused attention refers to an individual's ability to directly respond to particular visual, auditory, or tactile stimuli. The subscale includes number-oriented and text-oriented subtests in which participants identify a specific number and Chinese characters. Sustained attention refers to an individual's ability to maintain consistent behavioral responses during continuous and repetitive activities. This subscale includes petal comparison and digital circled subtests. Selective attention refers to an individual's ability to maintain action and cognition in the presence of external stimuli or fierce competition. This subscale includes a map search and symbol recognition subtests. Alternating attention is the ability of an individual to control attentional allocations with the mental flexibility to switch between dissimilar cognitive tasks. This subscale includes alternating symbols and a number of alternating subtests. Divided attention is the ability of an individual to respond appropriately to multiple tasks simultaneously. This subscale includes numerical and monophonic as well as pattern and monophonic detection subtests.

In terms of reliability, the scale scores were between 0.77 and 0.83 for the Cronbach α reliability coefficient, showing its good internal consistency. The test–retest reliability after four weeks was between 0.71 and 0.91. In terms of validity, the correlation between the full scale and each subtest was between 0.63 and 0.77 [29].

2.5. Statistical Analyses

Descriptive data of the measured variables are presented as mean and standard deviation (SD) or median and interquartile range (IQR, 25%–75% percentiles). The normality of study variables was examined with the Kolmogorov–Smirnov test. One-way analysis of variation (ANOVA) was used to analyze physical characteristics among the groups. A nonparametric test was used to compare all variables of the ASESC test based on the normality examination. The Kruskal–Wallis H test was used for between-group comparisons, whereas the Wilcoxon signed-rank test was used for within-group comparisons. Significant differences between the means or medians were set as $p < 0.05$. Additionally, Cohen's d effect size (ES) was used to quantify the magnitude of the training effect. The level of ES was defined as trivial (0.0–0.2), small (0.2–0.6), moderate (0.6–1.2), large (1.2–2.0), and very large (>2.0) [32]. Statistical analyses were conducted using SPSS® Statistics version 25.0 (IBM, Armonk, NY, USA) and Microsoft Excel 2016 (Microsoft Corporation, Redmond, WA, USA).

3. Results

3.1. Physical Characteristics

The physical characteristics of age, height, and body weight in all study groups are shown in Table 1.

Table 1. Physical characteristics of the participants.

		FIFA 11+ for Kids Boys (n = 13)	FIFA 11+ for Kids Girls (n = 13)	Control Boys (n = 13)	Control Girls (n = 13)	p-Value
Age (years)	Min	11.1	10.9	10.9	10.7	
	Max	11.7	11.6	11.7	11.7	
	Mean ± SD	11.4 ± 0.2	11.3 ± 0.2	11.3 ± 0.2	11.2 ± 0.4	p = 0.234
Height (cm)	Min	135.2	126.3	136.2	132.7	
	Max	162.2	155.7	148.7	154.6	
	Mean ± SD	146.1 ± 8.6	142.9 ± 8	141.2 ± 3.9	142.6 ± 6.6	p = 0.346
Weight (kg)	Min	26.4	25.1	28.7	23.3	
	Max	74.8	63.3	56.0	51.9	
	Mean ± SD	46.1 ± 14.4	38 ± 10.2	38 ± 7.5	34.4 ± 8.2	p = 0.045

Data are presented as minimum, maximum, and mean and standard deviation (Mean ± SD).

3.2. Attention Scales for Elementary School Children Test

As shown in Table 2, qualitative data of each ASESC item are analyzed with the Kruskal–Wallis H test for intergroup comparison and the Wilcoxon signed-rank test for intra-group comparison. For group comparisons, a significant difference was found in item 4 ($p < 0.019$), item 6 ($p = 0.038$), item 9 ($p = 0.019$), and item 10 ($p = 0.038$) of baseline assessment. In the post-training assessment, a significant difference was found in item 1 ($p < 0.001$), item 5 ($p < 0.001$), item 6 ($p < 0.001$), and item 7 ($p = 0.019$). Significant differences of pairwise comparisons between baseline and post-training assessments were identified in items 1, 2, 3, 4, and 5 for the training boys, items 1, 3, 4, 5, 6, and 7 for the training girls, items 3, 4, 6, and 9 for the control boys, and items 6 and 7 for the control girls ($p < 0.005$).

Table 2. The Attention Scale for Elementary School Children test items scores before and after the interventional period.

Variables	FIFA 11+ for Kids Boys (n = 13)				FIFA 11+ for Kids Girls (n = 13)				Control Boys (n = 13)				Control Girls (n = 13)				Baseline p-Value	Post-Test p-Value
	Baseline	Post-Test	MD	ES	Baseline	Post-Test	MD	ES	Baseline	Post-Test	MD	ES	Baseline	Post-Test	MD	ES		
Item 1	10.0 (7.0, 13.5)	14.0 (9.5, 15.0)*	−2.69	−0.64 (−1.45, 0.14)	9.0 (7.5, 11.5)	13.0 (11.0, 13.5)*	−3.15	−0.93 (−1.78, −0.14)	9.0 (8.0, 11.0)	9.0 (7.5, 11.0)	0.46	0.20 (−0.56, 0.98)	12.0 (9.5, 14.0)	11.0 (9.0, 13.0)	0.46	0.15 (−0.62, 0.92)	0.154	0.000 #
Item 2	9.0 (6.5, 11.5)	12.0 (10.0, 13.0)*	−3.15	−0.98 (−1.82, 0.18)	10.0 (6.5, 12.5)	12.0 (9.5, 14.0)	−2.23	−0.54 (−1.34, 0.23)	9.0 (7.5, 12.0)	10.0 (7.0, 12.0)	−0.46	−0.14 (−0.91, 0.63)	12.0 (9.5, 13.0)	10.0 (7.0, 11.0)	−0.46	−0.14 (−0.91, 0.63)	0.288	0.058
Item 3	10.0 (9.0, 11.0)	12.0 (10.0, 14.0)*	−2.08	−0.69 (−1.50, 0.09)	7.0 (3.5, 10.0)	11.0 (6.5, 15.0)*	−4.00	−0.97 (−1.81, −0.17)	9.0 (3.0, 11.5)	11.0 (9.0, 12.0)*	−2.00	−0.51 (−1.30, 0.26)	9.0 (6.5, 11.5)	11.0 (7.5, 12.0)	−2.00	−0.39 (−1.17, 0.38)	0.250	0.423
Item 4	12.0 (10.0, 13.0)	14.0 (12.5, 15.0)*	−2.31	−1.04 (−1.89, 0.23)	9.0 (5.0, 11.0)	10.0 (8.0, 14.0)*	−2.77	−0.80 (−1.62, −0.02)	9.0 (8.0, 11.5)	11.0 (9.0, 13.5)*	−1.85	−0.75 (−1.56, 0.03)	9.0 (7.0, 12.0)	9.0 (8.0, 14.0)	−1.85	−0.51 (−1.30, 0.27)	0.019 #	0.077
Item 5	15.0 (14.0, 17.0)	17.0 (16.0, 17.0)*	−0.92	−0.61 (−1.41, 0.16)	15.0 (14.0, 17.0)	17.0 (16.0, 17.0)*	−0.92	−0.85 (−1.68, −0.06)	17.0 (15.0, 17.0)	14.0 (12.0, 17.0)	2.31	1.08 (0.27, 1.93)	15.0 (12.0, 17.0)	15.0 (12.5, 17.0)	2.31	0.80 (0.01, 1.62)	0.269	0.000 #
Item 6	15.0 (13.0, 16.0)	16.0 (14.5, 17.5)	−0.46	−0.13 (−0.90, 0.64)	11.0 (8.5, 14.0)	15.0 (12.0, 16.5)*	−3.15	−0.86 (−1.69, −0.07)	14.0 (11.0, 15.5)	11.0 (10.0, 13.0)*	2.00	0.67 (−0.11, 1.48)	15.0 (14.0, 16.0)	12.0 (9.0, 13.0)*	2.00	0.51 (−0.27, 1.30)	0.038 #	0.000 #
Item 7	10.0 (9.0, 14.0)	14.0 (10.5, 14.5)	−1.77	0.48 (−1.27, 0.29)	9.0 (7.0, 12.5)	13.0 (11.0, 15.5)*	−3.23	−1.00 (−1.84, −0.20)	9.0 (7.0, 12.0)	10.0 (8.0, 12.0)	−0.62	−0.21 (−0.98, 0.56)	9.0 (4.0, 11.0)	10.0 (9.5, 13.5)*	−0.62	−0.20 (−0.97, 0.57)	0.712	0.019 #
Item 8	10.0 (8.5, 13.0)	11.0 (8.0, 14.5)	0.54	0.13 (−0.64, 0.90)	11.0 (7.0, 12.0)	11.0 (7.0, 13.5)	0.46	0.11 (−0.66, 0.88)	11.0 (7.0, 12.0)	8.0 (6.5, 9.0)	1.62	0.43 (−0.34, 1.22)	11.0 (4.5, 13.0)	9.0 (7.0, 10.0)	1.62	0.44 (−0.33, 1.23)	0.962	0.077
Item 9	12.0 (9.5, 14.0)	13.0 (11.0, 15.5)	−0.85	−0.25 (−1.03, 0.52)	9.0 (6.5, 12.5)	11.0 (7.5, 14.5)	−1.31	−0.33 (−1.11, 0.44)	9.0 (8.0, 11.0)	11.0 (9.5, 13.5)*	−1.62	−0.53 (−1.33, 0.24)	9.0 (7.5, 11.0)	11.0 (8.5, 13.0)	−1.62	−0.55 (−1.35, 0.22)	0.019 #	0.192
Item 10	12.0 (8.0, 13.5)	11.0 (7.0, 12.5)	0.92	0.26 (−0.51, 1.04)	8.0 (6.0, 11.5)	9.0 (6.0, 12.5)	−0.77	−0.21 (−0.98, 0.56)	11.0 (7.5, 12.5)	9.0 (4.0, 11.5)	1.31	0.33 (−0.43, 1.12)	8.0 (5.0, 11.0)	11.0 (5.5, 12.0)	1.31	0.41 (−0.36, 1.20)	0.038 #	0.750

Data are presented as median and interquartile (25–75%). Kruskal–Wallis H test was used for group comparison (significant difference indicated as #); Wilcoxon test was used for baseline and post-training comparison (significant difference indicated as *). n = number; MD = mean difference; ES = effect size.

In the total and subscales of the ASESC test (Figure 2), the Kruskal–Wallis H test demonstrates a significant difference in total scale, focused attention, selective attention, and alternating attention ($p < 0.001$). In comparing baseline and post-training assessments (the Wilcoxon signed-rank test), significant differences in pairwise comparison were found in total scale [$p < 0.001$, mean difference (MD) = −12.77, ES = 0.63], focused attention ($p < 0.001$, MD = −5.85, ES = −0.93), sustained attention ($p < 0.001$, MD = −4.38, ES = −1.14), and selective attention ($p = 0.019$, MD = −1.38, ES = −0.33) for the training boys; total scale ($p < 0.001$, MD = −17.15, ES = −0.90), focused attention ($p = 0.038$, MD = −5.15, ES = −0.96), sustained attention ($p < 0.001$, MD = −0.92, ES = −0.15), selective attention ($p < 0.001$, MD = −5.38, ES = −1.29), and divided attention ($p < 0.001$, MD = −0.77, ES = −0.12) for the training girls; sustained attention ($p < 0.001$, MD = −3.85, ES = −0.68) and selective attention for the control boys ($p < 0.001$, MD = 4.31, ES = 1.16); and focused attention ($p < 0.001$, MD = 2.92, ES = 0.58), sustain attention ($p = 0.019$, MD = −1.92, ES = −0.35), and selective attention ($p = 0.019$, MD = 3.31, ES = 0.56) for the control girls.

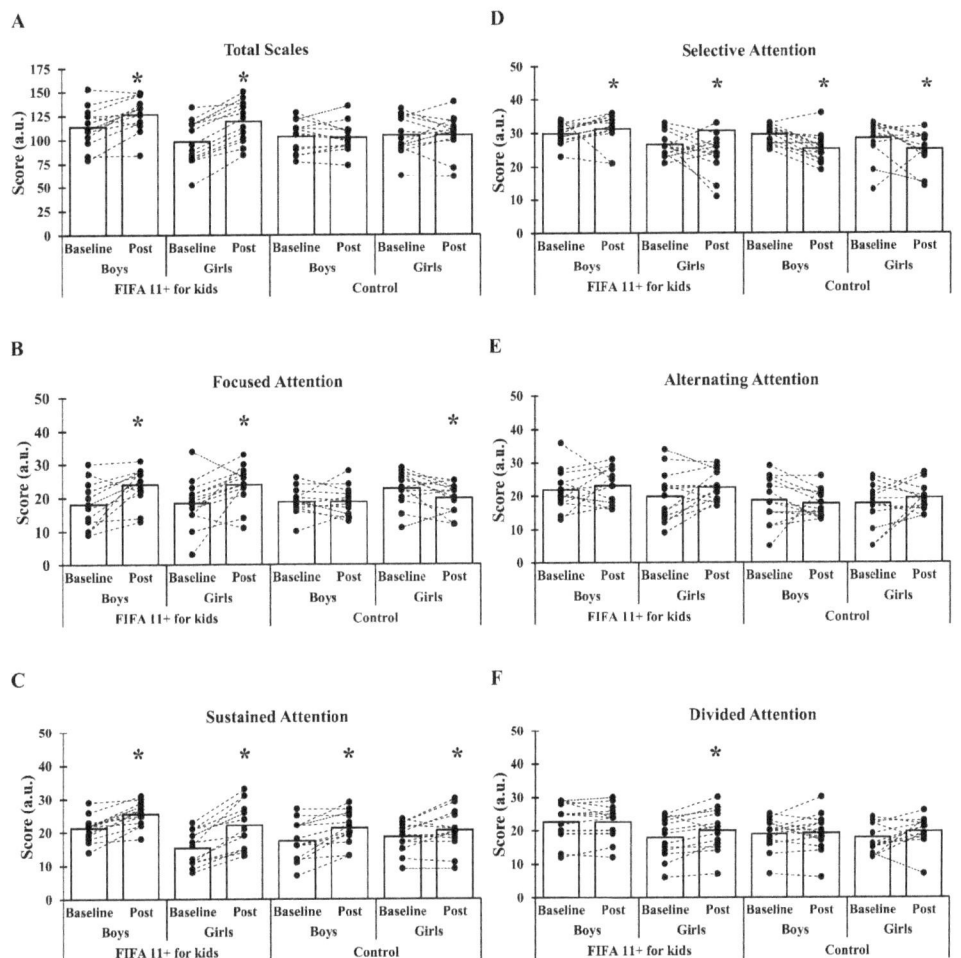

Figure 2. Pooled and individual subscales of the Attention Scale for Elementary School Children test before and after the interventional period in the FIFA 11+ for Kids boys, FIFA 11+ for Kids girls, control boys, and control girls; (**A**) total scale, (**B**) focused attention, (**C**) sustained attention, (**D**) selective attention, (**E**) alternating attention, and (**F**) divided attention. * indicates significant difference in the Wilcoxon test.

4. Discussion

As its first experimental initiative, the current study was designed to compare gender differences in attentional performances after an 8-week FIFA 11+ for Kids training intervention in elementary school children. Participants were assigned to two training groups who participated in the FIFA 11+ for Kids intervention and weekly PE lessons, and to two control groups who participated solely in weekly PE lessons. To achieve our research purpose, all children were invited to perform the ASESC test before and after the eight-week study period [29].

It is interesting to note that our results show significant increases in total scale, focused attention, sustained attention, and selective attention in both training groups, and divided attention solely in training girls. This finding demonstrated the positive effects of an 8-week structured exercise program on psychophysiological functions in processing focus-related cues in training children. The benefits of supplementary activities via the FIFA 11+ for Kids intervention on attentional capacities could be explained following the *"cardiovascular fitness hypothesis"* [33]. Accordingly, increased cardiovascular fitness, caused by regular physical activity adopted by an individual over time (i.e., longitudinal physical activity program over several weeks) is thought to improve angiogenesis [34] and neurogenesis [35] in areas of the brain that support memory and learning, subsequently enhancing cognitive performance [13,36]. As attention is a central mediator of cognition and learning performance [37,38], it is legitimate to suppose that an individual's attention capacities can be enhanced by participating in a supplementary chronic physical activity intervention (e.g., the FIFA 11+ for Kids program in the present study). Hence, the positive effects of an additional school-based program on attentional performances, as observed in the training boys and girls, could also be explained as following the *"cognitive stimulation hypothesis"* [39,40]. Indeed, the FIFA 11+ for Kids intervention could be classified as a cognitively engaging physical activity [28], as most exercises required attention, anticipation, and spatial orientation, particularly while engaged in dual-tasks [26]. Recently, some researchers have argued that chronic physical activities with a relatively high cognitive engagement (where children have to plan strategically and focus attention) have a larger effect on cognitive functions (including attentional capacity, problem solving, etc.) compared to simple physical activities intended to improve cardiovascular performance [20,28,41].

The second hypothesis in the present study assumed that training girls would benefit more from attentional improvement than training boys after the interventional period. This hypothesis could not be determined in focused, sustained, selective, and alternating attentions but it was identified in divided attention. Notably, we used numerical and monophonic, and pattern and monophonic detection subtests to evaluate divided attention in the present study. The children had to identify the right cues to achieve their tasks. It is interesting to note that divided attention is a type of simultaneous attention that allows an individual to synchronize different information cues and successfully carry out multiple tasks in the same period of time [42]. This evidence was supported by the poor capacity for divided attention observed in school children with ADHD [9]. Superior training adaptation regarding divided attention observed in girls could be related to gender differences in brain anatomy. It is well known that the female brain has a higher proportion of gray matter (densely packed with cell bodies), while the male brain has a higher proportion of white matter (consists of myelinated axons that form the connections between brain cells) in the prefrontal cortex [43,44]. In this context, Kanai and Rees [45] highlighted the important role of gray matter in attention. In fact, having more gray matter may explain why young women are usually more efficient at processing information, and usually excel at juggling several activities [46]. As a result, training girls profit more than boys from their participation in continual physical activity in terms of divided attention. It seems that long-term facilitation of the FIFA 11+ for Kids intervention could enhance attentional capacity in relation to multiple motor performance tasks in school children. This speculation was supported by the obtained results regarding divided attention in training and/or control girls groups.

Coincidently, participation in both control boys and girls significantly improved sustained attention. This finding indicated an increase in maintaining continuous and repetitive engagement. A possible explanation for this observation is related to daily routine regarding study activities and weekly engagements in school-based PE lessons after the winter vocation in the control groups. A review article conducted de Greeff et al. [36] reported that regular physical activities contribute positively to working memory, sustained attention, and academic performance in preadolescent children. As such, heathy children could possibly benefit their own sustained attention via regular school activities.

Several limitations of this study should be kept in mind, when interpreting the results. First, the small sample size may be a factor for the generalization of our results. This limitation is unavoidable because this investigation was carried out during the first wave of the COVID-19 pandemic in 2020, making it difficult for us to use a larger sample pool. Second, as a result of the same recruitment difficulties, we did not use a control group (inactive) in our experimental procedure. Third, the daily physical activities of both groups were not monitored during the study period. The lack of individual profiles of physical activities may potentially limit the interpretation of our research outcomes. Fourth, although the training children performed exercises according to the FIFA 11+ for Kids guidelines, individual variation in training intensity and involvement of group activities may be essential factors affecting training adaptation. Future studies should use tools to quantify training intensity (e.g., heart rate monitor or rating of perceived exertion). Lastly, the level of sexual maturation could be a potential factor influencing the attentional performance between boys and girls. Our findings were limited by the absence of biological examination to exclude the effects of age.

In the present study, attentional capacities were evaluated through convenient measurements. Further research is needed to explore brain adaptation regarding the positive effect of an 8-week FIFA 11+ for Kids intervention on attention in elementary school children. This can be performed through empirical measures, such as EEG or functional near-infrared spectroscopy (fNIRS).

5. Conclusions

In conclusion, the FIFA 11+ for Kids intervention is an effective school-based exercise for attentional improvement in schoolboys and girls. Facilitating an eight-week training program during the semester contributes to optimal performance in focused attention, sustained attention, and selective attention in year 5 schoolboys and girls. Likewise, schoolgirls show positive outcomes in divided attention after a supplementary exercise intervention on school days. The efficiency of the FIFA 11+ for Kids intervention for attentional adaptation in association with academic performance and psychometric health needs to be examined in future studies.

Author Contributions: Conceptualization, C.-H.C. and Y.-S.C.; methodology, C.-H.C. and Y.-S.C.; investigation, C.-H.C. and Y.-L.H. data curation, C.-H.C., G.R. and Y.B.; writing—original draft preparation, C.-H.C., G.R., Y.B., Y.-L.H. and Y.-S.C.; writing—review and editing, C.-H.C., G.R., Y.B. and Y.-S.C.; supervision, C.-H.C. and Y.-S.C.; project administration, C.-H.C. All authors have read and agreed to the published version of the manuscript.

Funding: This research received no external funding.

Institutional Review Board Statement: The study was conducted according to the guidelines of the Declaration of Helsinki, and approved by the Institutional Review Board of University of Taipei (protocol code UT-IRB-2020-003).

Informed Consent Statement: Informed consent was obtained from all the subjects involved in the study.

Data Availability Statement: The data are available upon request to the corresponding author via email.

Conflicts of Interest: No competing interest is reported for this study.

References

1. Posner, M.I.; Boies, S.J. Components of attention. *Psychol. Rev.* **1971**, *78*, 391–408. [CrossRef]
2. Posner, M.I.; Petersen, S.E. The attention system of the human brain. *Annu. Rev. Neurosci.* **1990**, *13*, 25–42. [CrossRef] [PubMed]
3. Fan, J.; Wu, Y.; Fossella, J.A.; Posner, M.I. Assessing the heritability of attentional networks. *BMC Neurosci.* **2001**, *2*, 14. [CrossRef]
4. Fossella, J.; Sommer, T.; Fan, J.; Wu, Y.; Swanson, J.M.; Pfaff, D.W.; Posner, M.I. Assessing the molecular genetics of attention networks. *BMC Neurosci.* **2002**, *3*, 14. [CrossRef]
5. Fan, J.; Fossella, J.A.; Summer, T.; Posner, M.I. Mapping the genetic variation of executive attention onto brain activity. *Proc. Natl. Acad. Sci. USA* **2003**, *100*, 7406–7411. [CrossRef] [PubMed]
6. Rueda, M.R.; Rothbart, M.K.; McCandliss, B.D.; Saccomanno, L.; Posner, M.I. Training, maturation, and genetic influences on the development of executive attention. *Proc. Natl. Acad. Sci. USA* **2005**, *102*, 14931–14936. [CrossRef] [PubMed]
7. McNab, F.; Varrone, A.; Farde, L.; Jucaite, A.; Bystritsky, P.; Forssberg, H.; Klingberg, T. Changes in cortical dopamine D1 receptor binding associated with cognitive training. *Science* **2009**, *323*, 800–802. [CrossRef] [PubMed]
8. Clarke, A.R.; Barry, R.J.; McCarthy, R.; Selikowitz, M. Age and sex effects in the EEG: Development of the normal child. *Clin. Neurophysiol.* **2001**, *112*, 806–814. [CrossRef]
9. Slobodin, O.; Davidovitch, M. Gender Differences in Objective and Subjective Measures of ADHD among Clinic-Referred Children. *Front. Hum. Neurosci.* **2019**, *13*, 441. [CrossRef]
10. Verburgh, L.; Königs, M.; Scherder, E.J.A.; Oosterlaan, J. Physical exercise and executive functions in preadolescent children, adolescents and young adults: A meta-analysis. *Br. J. Sports Med.* **2014**, *48*, 973–979. [CrossRef]
11. Chang, Y.K.; Labban, J.D.; Gapin, J.I.; Etnier, J.L. The effects of acute exercise on cognitive performance: A meta-analysis. *Brain Res.* **2012**, *1453*, 87–101. [CrossRef] [PubMed]
12. Audiffren, M. *Acute Exercise and Psychological Functions: A Cognitive Energetic Approach, in Exercise and Cognitive Function*, 1st ed.; McMorris, T., Tomporowski, P.D., Audiffren, M., Eds.; Wiley Online Library: Oxford, UK, 2009; pp. 3–39.
13. Etnier, J.L.; Salazar, W.; Landers, D.M.; Petruzzello, S.J.; Han, M.; Nowell, P. The influence of physical fitness and exercise upon cognitive functioning: A meta-analysis. *J. Sport Exerc. Psychol.* **1997**, *19*, 249–277. [CrossRef]
14. Tine, M.T.; Butler, A.G. Acute aerobic exercise impacts selective attention: An exceptional boost in lower-income children. *Educ. Psychol.* **2012**, *32*, 821–834. [CrossRef]
15. Hillman, C.H.; Pontifex, M.B.; Raine, L.B.; Castelli, D.M.; Hall, E.E.; Kramer, A.F. The effect of acute treadmill walking on cognitive control and academic achievement in preadolescent children. *Neuroscience* **2009**, *159*, 1044–1054. [CrossRef] [PubMed]
16. Sutoo, D.; Akiyama, K. Regulation of brain function by exercise. *Neurobiol. Dis.* **2003**, *13*, 1–14. [CrossRef]
17. Ferreira-Vieira, T.H.; Bastos, C.P.; Pereira, G.S.; Moreira, F.A.; Massensini, A.R. A role for the endocannabinoid system in exercise-induced spatial memory enhancement in mice. *Hippocampus* **2014**, *24*, 79–88. [CrossRef] [PubMed]
18. Mazzocco, M.M.; Kover, S.T. A longitudinal assessment of executive function skills and their association with math performance. *Child. Neuropsychol.* **2017**, *13*, 18–45. [CrossRef]
19. Gall, S.; Adams, L.; Joubert, N.; Ludyga, S.; Müller, I.; Nqweniso, S.; Pühse, U.; du Randt, R.; Seelig, H.; Smith, D.; et al. Effect of a 20-week physical activity intervention on selective attention and academic performance in children living in disadvantaged neighborhoods: A cluster randomized control trial. *PLoS ONE* **2018**, *13*, e0206908. [CrossRef] [PubMed]
20. Schmidt, M.; Jäger, K.; Egger, F.; Roebers, C.M.; Conzelmann, A. Cognitively engaging chronic physical activity, but not aerobic exercise, affects executive functions in primary school children: A group-randomized controlled trial. *J. Sport Exerc. Psychol.* **2015**, *37*, 575–591. [CrossRef]
21. Diamond, A. Close interrelation of motor development and cognitive development and of the cerebellum and prefrontal cortex. *Child. Dev.* **2000**, *71*, 44–56. [CrossRef]
22. Hsieh, S.S.; Lin, C.C.; Chang, Y.K.; Huang, C.J.; Hung, T.M. Effects of childhood gymnastics program on spatial working Memory. *Med. Sci. Sports Exerc.* **2017**, *49*, 2537–2547. [CrossRef]
23. Rössler, R.; Junge, A.; Bizzini, M.; Verhagen, E.; Chomiak, J.; Aus der Fünten, K.; Meyer, T.; Dvorak, J.; Lichtenstein, E.; Beaudouin, F.; et al. A multinational cluster randomised controlled trial to assess the efficacy of "11+ kids": A warm-up programme to prevent injuries in children's football. *Sports Med.* **2018**, *48*, 1493–1504. [CrossRef] [PubMed]
24. Rössler, R.; Verhagen, E.; Rommers, N.; Dvorak, J.; Junge, A.; Lichtenstein, E.; Donath, L.; Faude, O. Comparison of the "11+ Kids" injury prevention programme and a regular warm up in children's football (soccer): A cost effectiveness analysis. *Br. J. Sports Med.* **2019**, *53*, 309–314. [CrossRef] [PubMed]
25. Rössler, R.; Donath, L.; Bizzini, M.; Faude, O. A new injury prevention programme for children's football-FIFA 11+ Kids-can improve motor performance: A cluster-randomised controlled trial. *J. Sports Sci.* **2016**, *34*, 549–556. [CrossRef] [PubMed]
26. Pomares-Noguera, C.; Ayala, F.; Robles-Palazón, F.J.; Alomoto-Burneo, J.F.; López-Valenciano, A.; Elvira, J.L.L.; Hernández-Sánchez, S.; Croix, M.D.S. Training Effects of the FIFA 11+ Kids on Physical Performance in Youth Football Players: A Randomized Control Trial. *Front. Pediatr.* **2018**, *6*, 40. [CrossRef] [PubMed]
27. Zarei, M.; Abbasi, H.; Daneshjoo, A.; Gheitasi, M.; Johari, K.; Faude, O.; Rommers, N.; Rössler, R. The effect of the "11+ kids" on the isokinetic strength of young football players. *Int. J. Sports Physiol. Perform.* **2020**, *15*, 25–30. [CrossRef]
28. Tseng, W.Y.; Rekik, G.; Chen, C.H.; Clement, F.M.; Bezerra, P.; Crowley-McHattan, Z.; Chen, Y.S. Effects of 8-week FIFA 11+ for Kids intervention on physical fitness and attention in elementary school children. *J. Phys. Act. Health* **2021**, *18*, 686–693. [CrossRef]
29. Lin, H.Y.; Chou, T.J. The development of an attention test for elementary school children. *Bull. Spec. Educ.* **2010**, *35*, 29–53.

30. Sohlberg, M.M.; Mateer, C.A. Effectiveness of an attention training program. *J. Clin. Exp. Neuropsychol.* **1987**, *9*, 117–130. [CrossRef]
31. Sohlberg, M.M.; Mateer, C.A. Improving attention and managing attentional problems: Adapting rehabilitation techniques to adults with ADD. *Ann. N. Y. Acad. Sci.* **2001**, *931*, 359–375. [CrossRef]
32. Hopkins, W.G.; Marshall, S.W.; Batterham, A.M.; Hanin, J. Progressive statistics for studies in sports medicine and exercise science. *Med. Sci. Sport Exerc.* **2009**, *41*, 3–12. [CrossRef]
33. North, T.C.; McCullagh, P.; Tran, Z.V. Effect of exercise on depression. *Exerc. Sport Sci. Rev.* **1990**, *18*, 379–415. [CrossRef]
34. Isaacs, K.R.; Anderson, B.J.; Alcantara, A.A.; Black, J.E.; Greenough, W.T. Exercise and the brain: Angiogenesis in the adult rat cerebellum after vigorous physical activity and motor skill learning. *J. Cereb. Blood Flow Metab.* **1992**, *12*, 110–119. [CrossRef]
35. Dishman, R.K.; Berthoud, H.R.; Booth, F.W.; Cotman, C.W.; Edgerton, V.R.; Fleshner, M.R.; Gandevia, S.C.; Gomez-Pinilla, F.; Greenwood, B.N.; Hillman, C.H.; et al. Neurobiology of exercise. *Obesity* **2006**, *14*, 345–356. [CrossRef]
36. de Greeff, J.W.; Bosker, R.J.; Oosterlaan, J.; Visscher, C.; Hartman, E. Effects of physical activity on executive functions, attention and academic performance in preadolescent children: A meta-analysis. *J. Sci. Med. Sport* **2018**, *21*, 501–507. [CrossRef] [PubMed]
37. Hillman, C.H.; Snook, E.M.; Jerome, G.J. Acute cardiovascular exercise and executive control function. *Int. J. Psychophysiol.* **2003**, *48*, 307–314. [CrossRef]
38. Ison, M.S.; Greco, C.; Korzeniowski, C.G.; Morelato, G.S. Selective attention: A comparative study on Argentine students from different socioeconomic contexts. *Electron. J. Res. Educ. Psychol.* **2015**, *13*, 343–368. [CrossRef]
39. Tomporowski, P.D.; Davis, C.L.; Miller, P.H.; Naglieri, J.A. Exercise and children's intelligence, cognition, and academic achievement. *Educ. Psychol. Rev.* **2008**, *20*, 111–131. [CrossRef]
40. Pesce, C. Shifting the focus from quantitative to qualitative exercise characteristics in exercise and cognition research. *J. Sport Exerc. Psychol.* **2012**, *34*, 766–786. [CrossRef] [PubMed]
41. Vazou, S.; Pesce, C.; Lakes, K.; Smiley-Oyen, A. More than one road leads to Rome: A narrative review and meta-analysis of physical activity intervention effects on cognition in youth. *Int. J. Sport Exerc. Psychol.* **2019**, *17*, 153–178. [CrossRef] [PubMed]
42. Spelke, E.; Hirst, W.; Neisser, U. Skills of divided attention. *Cognition* **1976**, *4*, 215–230. [CrossRef]
43. Gur, R.C.; Turetsky, B.I.; Matsui, M.; Yan, M.; Bilker, W.; Hughett, P.; Gur, R.E. Sex differences in brain gray and white matter in healthy young adults: Correlations with cognitive performance. *J. Neurosci.* **1999**, *19*, 4065–4072. [CrossRef]
44. Solianik, R.; Brazaitis, M.; Skurvydas, A. Sex-related differences in attention and memory. *Medicina* **2016**, *52*, 372–377. [CrossRef]
45. Kanai, R.; Rees, G. The structural basis of inter-individual differences in human behaviour and cognition. *Nat. Rev. Neurosci.* **2011**, *12*, 231–242. [CrossRef]
46. Van Schouwenburg, M.R.; Onnink, A.M.H.; Ter Huurne, N.; Kan, C.C.; Zwiers, M.P.; Hoogman, M.; Franke, B.; Buitelaar, J.K.; Cools, R. Cognitive flexibility depends on white matter microstructure of the basal ganglia. *Neuropsychologia* **2014**, *53*, 171–177. [CrossRef]

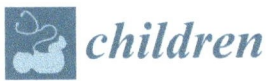

Article

The Effects of Exercise Difficulty and Time-of-Day on the Perception of the Task and Soccer Performance in Child Soccer Players

Liwa Masmoudi [1,2], Adnene Gharbi [1], Cyrine H'Mida [1,2], Khaled Trabelsi [1,2], Omar Boukhris [1,3], Hamdi Chtourou [1,3], Mohamed Amine Bouzid [1,2], Cain C. T. Clark [4], Nizar Souissi [1,3], Thomas Rosemann [5] and Beat Knechtle [5,6,*]

1. Institut Supérieur du Sport et de l'éducation Physique de Sfax, Université de Sfax, Sfax 3000, Tunisia; liwa.masmoudi@yahoo.fr (L.M.); adnenegharbi@yahoo.fr (A.G.); sirinehmida7@gmail.com (C.H.); trabelsikhaled@gmail.com (K.T.); omarboukhris24@yahoo.com (O.B.); h_chtourou@yahoo.fr (H.C.); mohamedamine.bouzid@isseps.usf.tn (M.A.B.); n_souissi@yahoo.fr (N.S.)
2. Research Laboratory: Education, Motricité, Sport et Santé, EM2S, LR19JS01, High Institute of Sport and Physical Education of Sfax, University of Sfax, Sfax 3000, Tunisia
3. Activité Physique, Sport et Santé, UR18JS01, Observatoire National du Sport, Tunis 1003, Tunisia
4. Centre for Intelligent Healthcare, Coventry University, Coventry CV1 5FB, UK; ad0183@coventry.ac.uk
5. Institute of Primary Care, University of Zurich, 8006 Zurich, Switzerland; thomas.rosemann@usz.ch
6. Medbase St. Gallen Am Vadianplatz, 9000 St. Gallen, Switzerland
* Correspondence: beat.knechtle@hispeed.ch

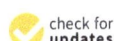

Citation: Masmoudi, L.; Gharbi, A.; H'Mida, C.; Trabelsi, K.; Boukhris, O.; Chtourou, H.; Bouzid, M.A.; Clark, C.C.T.; Souissi, N.; Rosemann, T.; et al. The Effects of Exercise Difficulty and Time-of-Day on the Perception of the Task and Soccer Performance in Child Soccer Players. *Children* 2021, 8, 793. https://doi.org/10.3390/children8090793

Academic Editor: Zoe Knowles

Received: 31 July 2021
Accepted: 7 September 2021
Published: 10 September 2021

Publisher's Note: MDPI stays neutral with regard to jurisdictional claims in published maps and institutional affiliations.

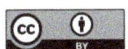

Copyright: © 2021 by the authors. Licensee MDPI, Basel, Switzerland. This article is an open access article distributed under the terms and conditions of the Creative Commons Attribution (CC BY) license (https://creativecommons.org/licenses/by/4.0/).

Abstract: In soccer, accurate kicking skills are important determinants of successful performance. A successful kick must meet several criteria, including speed, accuracy, and timing. In fact, players who are able to kick the ball more accurately under various difficulties, such as time pressure, space constraints, the opponent's pressure, and the distance between the kicking point and the goal, have a clear advantage during soccer games. The aim of the present study was to investigate the effect of exercise difficulty and time-of-day on perceived task difficulty and kicking performance. Accordingly, 32 boys (age: 11 ± 0.7 years; height: 1.45 ± 0.07 m; body-mass: 38.9 ± 7.8 kg) performed shooting accuracy tests under two difficulty levels (distance (long-distance (LD) vs. short-distance (SD)) and time pressure (Without-time-pressure (WTP) vs. With-time-pressure (TP)) at 08:00 h and 17:00 h. Absolute-error, variable-error, and constant-error were evaluated during the kicking tasks, in addition to ball velocity and shooting quality. Moreover, rating-of-perceived-exertion score (RPE), feeling-scale (FS), and perceived difficulty were completed immediately at the end of each test. The results showed that shooting quality was not affected by the time-of-day, but it was better in WTP vs. TP ($p < 0.05$), and in SD vs. LD ($p < 0.05$), respectively. Higher values for FS and lower values for RPE were observed in the morning compared to the afternoon ($p < 0.05$) and in WTP vs. TP ($p < 0.05$). In conclusion, specific soccer skills of boys were not time-of-day dependent, but they may be associated with time pressure and task difficulty.

Keywords: perceived difficulty; psychomotor performance; diurnal variation; child; mood; soccer

1. Introduction

The influence of time-of-day effects on psycho-physiological, cognitive, and physical performance assessments has been widely studied [1]. Indeed, in children, previous studies have reported that muscle power [2], strength [3], agility [4], and aerobic fitness [2,5,6] were better at the end of the afternoon compared to the morning hours. Likewise, some psycho-physiological functions, such as cardiovascular and metabolic responses to exercise [7], mental [6], psychomotor [8], and cognitive performances [9–11] have been found to be better in the late afternoon, approximately corresponding to the circadian peak of body temperature [4,12]. However, contrastingly, Huguet et al. [13] reported that several simple coordination skills tend to peak earlier in the day compared to complex coordinative skills [13]. Discrepancies between the findings reported in the literature could be related to differences in the mental load of the task, the type of the task, and the perceived difficulty.

In this context, Elghoul et al. [9,10] investigated the time-of-day effects on dart-throwing performance from short and long distance and the perception of the difficulty of the task. Accordingly, the authors reported better performance in both long and short distance at 17:00 h compared to 07:00 h, concomitant to significant reductions in perceived task difficulty from 07:00 h to 17:00 h.

Pertaining to the previous studies, a number of limitations may be manifest related to the chosen task and method employed. Moreover, the number of participants for these studies was small, precluding any firm conclusions. Furthermore, assessment of accuracy was performed across a number of points using different protocols (i.e., scores per trial, numbers of zeros scored, radial error); indeed, this method of accuracy estimation is inadequate and presents low reliability [14]. It has been posited that the direct measures, such as the absolute error, variable error, and constant error, as well as velocity (the kicked object) could provide both a more valid and more informative description of the kicking performance [14].

Goal scoring is an important element in soccer [15] that necessitates, particularly during key moments of the match-play, high velocity and accuracy of shooting. Indeed, previous studies have reported a direct relationship between speed of leg movement and subsequent ball speed [16]. However, it should be acknowledged that an increased execution speed can deleteriously affect accuracy [17]. In goal-directed aiming tasks, increased time pressure and increased target distance will impact the index of difficulty [18]. Therefore, shooting at a target under time-pressured conditions, in response to the demanding nature of competitive soccer, would conceivably elicit an increased execution speed and, in turn, a decreased accuracy. Indeed, previous studies addressing instep kicks have proven that, by prioritizing accuracy, the ball kicking velocity can be significantly reduced [19]. Moreover, in children, Frikha et al. [20] found that the instep kicking accuracy and missed kicks were significantly decreased in time-pressured vs. free conditions. In addition, the perception of difficulty was higher in time-pressured vs. free conditions [20].

A dearth of studies has investigated the effects of time-of-day on coordination skills in soccer [4,12]. Of the available data, some studies reported that kicking accuracy, juggling performance, ball control with the body, and ball control with the head were not affected by the time-of-day [4,12]. However, other investigations showed that coordination skills of kicking accuracy, juggling, and dribbling performance were better in the afternoon compared to the morning [6,21].

Indeed, little is known about the association of circadian rhythms and level of difficulty. Moreover, the diurnal variation of coordination skill performance in children remains scarcely investigated. Therefore, we hypothesized that kicking accuracy would be better without time pressure (WTP) compared to time-pressure (TP) and for the short compared to the long distance. In addition, we hypothesized that psychomotor performance would be better in the afternoon compared to the morning hours. Accordingly, the aim of this study was to examine the effect of time-of-day (08:00 h and 17:00 h) and the level of difficultly (kicking WTP and kicking TP conditions from a long (10 m) and a short (6 m) distance) on kicking accuracy and perceived difficulty in child soccer players.

2. Materials and Methods

2.1. Participants

Thirty-two male soccer players (age: 11 ± 0.7 years; height: 1.45 ± 0.07 m [WHO Z-score = 0.03]; body-mass: 38.9 ± 7.8 kg [WHO Z-score = 0.75]; body mass index: 18.5 kg/m^2 [WHO Z-score = 0.74]), from three teams of the first division Tunisian youth league, voluntarily participated in the study. They participated in four training sessions per week and one match at the weekend (usually on Sunday). All boys were classified as prepubertal (stage 1) by a pediatrician, according to Tanner criteria [22]. Participants were included in the present study if: (a) his age was between 10 and 12 years, (b) he had no history of neurological, musculoskeletal, or orthopedic disorders or had no history of lower extremity surgery or injury in the 6 months before testing that might have affected their physical ability, (c) he was able to understand and follow instructions, and (d) he had no cognitive or visual problems.

Before participation to the study, boys and their parents/guardians provided written informed consent, and they were informed that they could withdraw from the study at any time.

2.2. Procedure

After two familiarization sessions, boys performed a shooting accuracy tests (10 kicks) on a target of 1.2 m radius, under two difficulty levels (distance and time pressure). First, they performed the test from two distances: 6 m and 10 m. The distances of 6 m and 10 m were chosen arbitrarily to reflect short and long distances, respectively [23]. Second, to increase the difficulty level of the task for each distance, boys were instructed to complete the 10 kicks as accurately as possible, WTP and TP. During TP, the boys were asked to perform the test shot with a frequency of 1 shot every 3 s and during WTP they were asked to perform the test shot with a frequency of 1 shot every 6 s. The frequency of the shots was controlled by an audible signal emitted by an audio source.

The measurements were taken, in a randomized order, at two different time-of-day: 08:00 h and 17:00 h. For each test session, boys woke up at 06h30 and ate a standardized breakfast. At 12h30, boys ate a standardized iso-caloric lunch. From 12h30 onward, boys were allowed to consume only drinking water. At the beginning of each test session, boys were asked to complete the Profile of Mood States (POMS) questionnaire. In addition, intra-aural temperature (ThermoScan IRT 4520, Braun GmbH, Kronberg, Germany), heart rate (Polar Team System, Polar Electro Oy, Kempele, Finland), and systolic (SBP) and diastolic (DBP) blood pressure (Beurer, B.M 20, 89077 Ulm, Germany) were measured at the beginning of each session. Moreover, the boys indicated their rating of perceived exertion (RPE), feeling scale (FS), and perceived task difficulty (PD), immediately at the end of the kicking test (Figure 1).

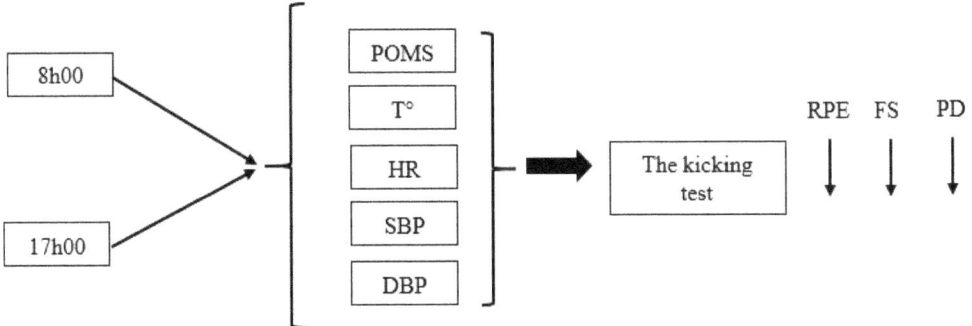

Figure 1. Schematic representation of the experimental design. POMS: Profile of mood states; T°: temperature; HR: heart rate; SBP: systolic blood pressure; DBP: diastolic blood pressure; RPE: rating of perceived exertion; FS: feeling scale; PD: perceived task difficulty.

2.3. Kicking Accuracy

The kicking accuracy test consisted of performing 10 kicks from a point placed at 6 and 10 m from the target, respectively [23]. To determine the accuracy of the kick, we analyzed video recordings of each trial. Absolute error (AE), variable error (VE), and constant error (CE) were evaluated as the variables of kicking accuracy (Figure 2). Further, ball velocity

(BV; measured via radar gun), and shooting quality (SQ; shooting accuracy divided by the time elapsed from hitting the ball to the bulls-eye) were determined.

2.4. Perceived Exertion Scale Rating

The RPE measure was obtained based on the Borg's category ratio-scale (CR-10), as modified by Foster et al. [24]. Boys rated how hard the exercise felt from a scale of 0 (nothing at all) to 10 (maximal). The RPE scale is a reliable indicator of physical discomfort, has sound psychometric properties, and is strongly correlated with several other physiological measures of exertion [24].

2.5. Feeling Scale

Affect was measured using a FS [25]. The FS items were rated on an 11-point scale: +5, very good; +3, good; +1, fairly good; 0, neutral; −1, fairly bad; −3, bad; −5, very bad. The scale was used to measure the affective component of exercise, i.e., whether the exercise felt pleasant or unpleasant.

2.6. Perceived Difficulty

PD was assessed according to the difficulty perception −15 scale [26], a 15-points category scale, with 7 labels, from "extremely easy" to "extremely difficult", symmetrically placed around a central label, "somewhat difficult".

2.7. The Profile of Mood States (POMS)

The POMS is a self-report questionnaire, developed by McNair [27], including 65 items, measuring five negative moods (tension-anxiety, depression, anger-hostility, vigor-activity, fatigue, and confusion-bewilderment), one positive mood (vigor), and interpersonal relationships, and a total mood disturbance score (TMD). Five-point Likert scales, ranging from 0 ("not at all") to 4 ("extreme") were used.

$$TMD = (Tension + Depression + Anger + Fatigue + Confusion) - Vigor$$

2.8. Statistical Analysis

All statistical tests were processed using STATISTICA software (StatSoft, version 12, Paris, France). All values were expressed as mean ± SD. G*power software (version 3.1.9.2; Kiel University, Kiel, Germany) [28] was used to calculate the required sample size. Values for α were set at 0.05 and power at 0.8. Based on the study of Masmoudi et al. [12] and consensus between the authors, the effect size was estimated to be 0.49. Accordingly, the required sample size for this study was 28. Following normality confirmation using the Kolmogorov-Smirnov test, the data of the kicking accuracy variables (AE, VE, CE, BV, SQ), FS, RPE, and PD were analyzed using a three-way repeated measure analysis of variance (ANOVA) (2 conditions (WTP and TP) × 2 distances (SD and LD) × 2 time-of-day (08:00 h and 17:00 h), and, when appropriate, Bonferroni post-hoc tests were used to determine where significant differences existed. In addition, partial eta-squared (η_p^2) was calculated for these variables. Finally, differences in temperature, HR, SBP, DBP, and POMS were compared using paired-sample t-tests. Statistical significance was set, a priori, at $p < 0.05$.

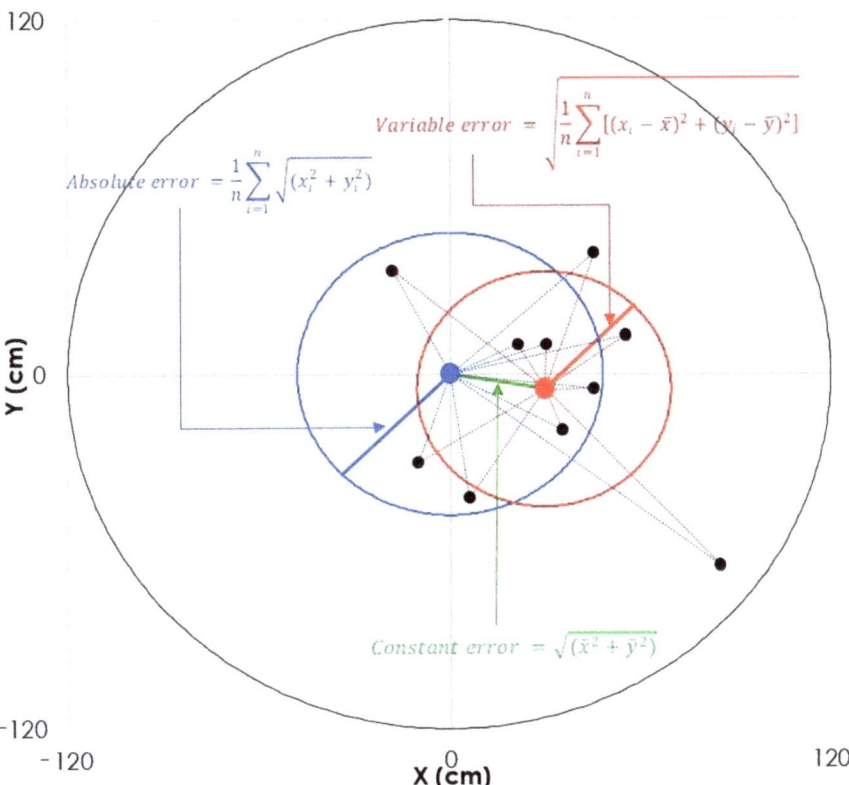

Figure 2. Schematic representation of the ten bullet impact points with the target and the three accuracy errors. The large black circle represents the target (1.2 m radius); The blue point represents the center of the target; The ten black dots represent the points of impact of the ball with the target; Blue dashed lines represent absolute errors; The radius of the blue circle represents the mean absolute error of the 10 shots; The red point represents the barycenter of the 10 black points; Red dashed lines represent relative errors; The radius of the red circle represents the average relative error of the 10 shots; The green line represents the constant error.

3. Results

3.1. Psychomotor Parameters

3.1.1. Kicking Accuracy

The 3-way ANOVA on AE indicated significant main effects of condition ($F_{(1,31)} = 103.48$; $p < 0.001$, $\eta_p^2 = 0.769$) and distance ($F_{(1,31)} = 276.72$; $p < 0.001$; $\eta_p^2 = 0.899$); no significant main effect for time-of-day or significant interactions were found.

The Bonferroni post hoc test revealed that AE with WTP and TP was significantly lower in SD compared to LD ($p < 0.001$), and AE during SD and LD was higher for TP compared to WTP ($p < 0.001$) (Table 1).

The variable error revealed the same main effects for condition ($F_{(1,31)} = 8.63$; $p < 0.006$, $\eta_p^2 = 0.218$) and distance ($F_{(1,31)} = 121.02$; $p < 0.001$; $\eta_p^2 = 0.796$), without a significant main effect for time-of-day or significant interactions between these variables.

The Bonferroni post hoc test revealed that the variable error with WTP and TP was significantly lower in SD compared to LD ($p < 0.001$) (Table 1).

The CE revealed only a significant main effect for distance ($F_{(1,31)} = 21.91$; $p < 0.001$, $\eta_p^2 = 0.414$).

The Bonferroni post hoc test revealed that CE, with TP at only 17h00, was significantly lower in SD compared to LD ($p = 0.007$) (Table 1).

Table 1. Kicking accuracy and velocity, perceived difficulty, feeling score, and rating of perceived exertion (RPE) recorded at 08:00 h and 17:00 h during the short (SD) and long (LD) distances for the two experimental conditions (without time pressure (WTP) and with time pressure (TP)).

Variable		WTP		TP	
		SD	LD	SD	LD
Absolute error (cm)	08:00 h	53.5 ± 12.7	79.1 ± 12.5 [1]	67.9 ± 13.6 [2]	93.3 ± 10.3 [1,2]
	17:00 h	53.8 ± 13.2	76.8 ± 14.3 [1]	65.9 ± 16.8 [2]	91.8 ± 10.5 [1,2]
Variable error (cm)	08:00 h	47.9 ± 12	67.1 ± 13.7 [1]	50.1 ± 13.1	71.9 ± 13.3 [1]
	17:00 h	50.7 ± 13.7	67.7 ± 14.4 [1]	52.1 ± 17.2	72.4 ± 11.3 [1]
Constant error (cm)	08:00 h	19.6 ± 14.8	27.7 ± 16.4	22.5 ± 16.1	29.1 ± 15.5
	17:00 h	18.7 ± 12.6	28.7 ± 14.9	21 ± 9.1	32 ± 17.3 [1]
Ball velocity (m/s)	08:00 h	9.6 ± 1.3	10.5 ± 1.7 [1]	8.7 ± 1.2	9.1 ± 1.4
	17:00 h	9.6 ± 1.4	10.5 ± 1.6 [1]	8.7 ± 1.7	9.2 ± 1.3
Shooting quality (m/s)	08:00 h	1.06 ± 0.25	0.43 ± 0.14 [1]	0.75 ± 0.22 [2]	0.24 ± 0.1 [1,2]
	17:00 h	0.85 ± 0.22	0.8 ± 0.17 [1]	0.96 ± 0.29 [2]	0.84 ± 0.14 [1,2]
Perceived difficulty (A.U)	08:00 h	4.84 ± 2.33	6.31 ± 1.97 [1]	5.03 ± 2.61	5.81 ± 2.31 [1]
	17:00 h	5.56 ± 2.68	6.47 ± 2.63	4.75 ± 2.37	7.03 ± 2.75 [1]
Feeling score (A.U)	08:00 h	2.19 ± 2.62	2.28 ± 1.53	3.16 ± 1.92 [2]	3.34 ± 2.22 [2]
	17:00 h	3.19 ± 1.8 [3]	2.09 ± 1.49 [1]	2.69 ± 1.71	0.63 ± 1.68 [1,2,3]
RPE (A.U)	08:00 h	1.0 ± 1.02	1.16 ± 0.88 [1]	0.78 ± 1.16	1.63 ± 1.62 [1]
	17:00 h	1.03 ± 1.18	1.34 ± 0.6	1.5 ± 1.34 [3]	2.16 ± 1.14 [2,3]

[1]: Significantly different compared to SD at $p < 0.05$; [2]: Significantly different compared to WTP at $p < 0.05$; [3]: Significantly different compared to 08:00 h at $p < 0.05$.

3.1.2. Kicking Velocity

The 3-way ANOVA on ball velocity indicated significant main effects of condition ($F_{(1,31)} = 61.26$; $p < 0.001$, $\eta_p^2 = 0.664$) and distance: $F_{(1,31)} = 21.11$; $p < 0.001$; $\eta_p^2 = 0.405$); but no main significant effect for time-of-day or significant interactions were found.

The Bonferroni post hoc test revealed that the ball velocity with WTP was significantly lower in SD compared to LD ($p < 0.05$) (Table 1).

For shooting quality, we found significant main effects for condition ($F_{(1,31)} = 101.25$; $p < 0.001$, $\eta_p^2 = 0.766$) and distance ($F_{(1,31)} = 532.6$; $p < 0.001$; $\eta_p^2 = 0.945$). In addition, the results showed a significant condition × distance interaction ($F_{(1,31)} = 6.25$; $p < 0.05$, $\eta_p^2 = 0.168$). The Bonferroni post hoc testing revealed that shooting quality with SD was significantly better in WTP compared to TP ($p < 0.001$), and that shooting quality during TP was better for SD compared to LD ($p < 0.001$) (Table 1).

3.2. Perceived Difficulty and Psychological Parameters

For FS, the results showed significant main effects for time-of-day ($F_{(1,31)} = 10.41$; $p = 0.003$, $\eta_p^2 = 0.251$) and distance ($F_{(1,31)} = 8.03$; $p < 0.01$; $\eta_p^2 = 0.206$). In addition, significant interactions time-of-day × condition ($F_{(1,31)} = 33.49$; $p < 0.001$, $\eta_p^2 = 0.519$) and time-of-day × distance ($F_{(1,31)} = 12.31$; $p < 0.001$, $\eta_p^2 = 0.284$) were observed. The Bonferroni post hoc testing revealed that FS score was higher in TP at 08:00 h than 17:00 h ($p < 0.001$) and that FS score in TP was higher than WTP at 08:00 h ($p < 0.001$) and at 17:00 h ($p < 0.01$), respectively (Table 1). The FS score for the LD condition at 17:00 h was significantly lower than at 08:00 h ($p < 0.001$) and was lower during LD compared to SD in the two time-of-day ($p < 0.001$) (Table 1).

The PD was not affected by the time-of-day and time pressure. However, a significant main effect for distance ($F_{(1,31)} = 34.67$; $p < 0.001$, $\eta_p^2 = 0.528$) was observed. PD score was higher in LD compared to SD ($p < 0.001$). POMS subscale, TMD scores, and t-test results at the two measurements are presented in Table 2. The depression and the vigor scores were significantly higher at 17:00 h compared to 08:00 h ($p < 0.05$). However, anger, confusion, fatigue, inter-relation, and the TMD scores were not significantly affected by the time-of-day (Table 2).

Table 2. The POMS subscale and TMD scores recorded at the two times of day.

Variable	08:00 h	17:00 h	t-Test	p-Value
Anxiety (A.U)	2.6 ± 3.1	3.2 ± 3.7	0.69	0.496
Anger (A.U)	5.5 ± 4	5 ± 5.2	0.43	0.669
Confusion (A.U)	2.1 ± 3.7	2 ± 2.2	0.12	0.905
Depression (A.U)	1.6 ± 2.1	3.1 ± 4.2	2.47	0.019
Fatigue (A.U)	2.3 ± 2.7	2.3 ± 3.2	0.06	0.955
Vigor (A.U)	26 ± 4.3	28.1 ± 4.2	2.19	0.036
Interpersonal-Relationship (A.U)	23.1 ± 5	23.3 ± 4.4	0.12	0.908
TMD (A.U)	−12.1 ± 11.8	−12.5 ± 18.2	0.13	0.896

Concerning RPE, our results showed a significant main effects for time-of-day ($F_{(1,31)} = 21.41$; $p < 0.001$; $\eta_p^2 = 0.408$), condition ($F_{(1,31)} = 18.46$; $p < 0.001$; $\eta_p^2 = 0.373$), and distance ($F_{(1,31)} = 14.51$; $p < 0.001$; $\eta_p^2 = 0.319$). The statistical analysis revealed higher RPE scores (i) at 17:00 h than 08:00 h (Table 1) ($p < 0.05$) and (ii) during LD and TP compared to SD and WTP, respectively ($p < 0.05$ and $p < 0.05$) (Table 2).

3.3. Physiological Parameters

Statistical analysis showed that intra-aural temperature and HR values were significantly higher at 17:00 h than 08:00 h (+ 3.4%, $p < 0.001$ and + 4.7%, $p < 0.05$, respectively, Table 3). However, no significant time-of-day effect was found for systolic and diastolic blood pressures (Table 3).

Table 3. Intra-oral temperature, heart rate (HR), systolic blood pressure (SBP) and diastolic blood pressure (DBP) recorded at the two time-of-day.

Variable	08:00 h	17:00 h	t-Test	p-Value
Temperature (°C)	35 ± 0.8	36.2 ± 0.5	7.46	<0.001
HR (b·min^{-1})	84 ± 9	88 ± 11	2.26	0.031
SBP (mmHg)	11.4 ± 0.7	11.5 ± 1.1	0.21	0.833
DBP (mmHg)	6.5 ± 0.7	6.6 ± 1.2	0.33	0.741

4. Discussion

The principal findings of the current study were (i) there was no significant time-of-day differences between 08:00 h and 17:00 h regarding kicking accuracy, (ii) kicking accuracy was higher without vs. with time pressure, (iii) feelings scale scores were greater in the morning vs. afternoon, and during SD vs. LD at 17h00, respectively, (iv) the RPE scores were higher during TP vs. WTP, and in the afternoon vs. the morning, respectively, and (v) the RPE scores were higher during LD vs. SD in TP, and TP vs. WTP in the LD condition, respectively.

The current study suggested that specific soccer skills of boys are not dependent on time-of-day. In line with the present study, Gharbi et al. [4] noted that soccer skills of boys did not differ between 07:00 h and 17:00 h. Indeed, the authors reported that, in Tunisian boys (mean age: 12.7 years), kicking accuracy and juggling performance remained unaffected by time-of-day. Similarly, Masmoudi et al. [12], in Tunisian children (mean age: 14.6 years), concluded that shooting accuracy was not impacted by time-of-day. However, some other soccer specific skills have been reported to be time-of-day dependent [4,12]. In this context, Gharbi et al. [4] showed that agility and dribbling were better in the afternoon vs. the morning; whilst Masmoudi et al. [12] concurred with this finding and reported that dribbling performance was better at 13:00 h and 17:00 h vs. 08:00 h. In this context, it has been reported that the diurnal rhythm of intra-aural temperature could explain the diurnal variation of dribbling performance [12]. In fact, the increase in intra-aural temperature in the afternoon could enhance the conduction velocity of the action potentials as well as metabolic reactions, improving muscle contraction during the dribbling test. However, although intra-aural temperature values were significantly higher at 17:00 h than 08:00 h, there were no significant time-of-day differences between 08:00 h and 17:00 h for the kicking accuracy. Therefore, the present study indicates that technical specific skills (i.e., kicking accuracy) is not associated with the diurnal rhythm of intra-aural temperature. It is difficult to explain these discrepancies between studies pertaining to diurnal variation of soccer specific skills in children; however, it is possible that dribbling performance is related, at least in part, to the sprint and agility qualities that have been shown to be better in the afternoon [4,12]. Accordingly, Bernard et al. [29] reported that sprint performance was time-of-day dependent, with better outcomes in the afternoon compared to the morning. Similarly, other short-term maximal performances (e.g., vertical jump, repeated sprints, etc.) have been shown to be better in the afternoon vs. morning [2,3,5,30]. It is conceivable, as shown in the present results, that technical specific skills (i.e., kicking accuracy) of soccer players are not affected by the time-of-day of testing; however, when technical skills are coupled with physical abilities (e.g., agility, dribbling, etc.), significant diurnal variation of children' performances may be observed.

The lack of a significant time-of-day effect on kicking accuracy could be, at least partly, related to the typical time-of-day of training (i.e., soccer training sessions in the academy that took place in the morning hours). Indeed, in boys, Souissi et al. [3] noted that regular training in the morning hours could significantly affect the diurnal variation of short-term maximal performance. Given that boys recruited for the present study regularly trained in the morning hours, we could speculate that this training adaptation could, partially, explain the non-significant time-of-day effect on kicking accuracy. Likewise, better feelings scores in the morning (i.e., the reported time-of-day of worse performance) were observed, which could indicate that boys prefer performing tests in the morning hours, as they regularly trained at this time-of-day, and this could improve their performance and affect the normal diurnal variation of performance. This suggests that a lower psychological discomfort reported in the morning could have contributed to the better performance reported in that time-of-day. In support of this idea, the TMD scores were not significantly affected by the time-of-day, which could explain the lack of a significant time-of-day effect on kicking accuracy. In this context, we also showed that RPE scores were higher in the afternoon hours (indicating higher physiological discomfort in the afternoon vs. morning), which could suggest that boys in the present study were better prepared to perform the tests in the morning hours. In addition, the higher motivation of participants in the morning could explain also the previously reported morning to afternoon difference. Likewise, HR values were higher at 17:00 h than 08:00 h. The higher values of RPE and HR in the afternoon hours could be related to the amount of activity undertaken in the afternoon by children. Additionally, the PD was not affected by the time-of-day, which could also explain the lack of a significant time-of-day effect on kicking accuracy. Indeed, PD mainly reflects the amount of resources, or effort, that boys have devoted to the task in order to reach a given level of performance [9]. In fact, it has been shown that, in children, fatigue during testing of soccer-specific skills is not affected by the time-of-day [12]. Furthermore, SBP and DBP did not vary with time-of-day, which could explain why specific soccer skills of boys were not time-of-day dependent.

For task difficulty, the present study showed that performance was better WTP in comparison to TP. To the best of our knowledge, this is the first study examining the effect of time-pressure on kicking accuracy in boys according to different times-of-day. During a dart-throwing task, Elghoul et al. [9,10] investigated the task difficulty at 07:00 h and 17:00 h, and reported that the PD was higher with LD vs. SD due to geometry. However, in the present study, we did not report a significant time-of-day effect on PD. The discrepancies between the findings of the present study and those of Elghoul et al. [9,10] could be related to the utilized psychomotor task (kicking accuracy (coordination visual perception and lower body) vs. dart-throwing (coordination visual perception and upper body)). The effect of PD on psychomotor performance should be interpreted with caution because PD was measured immediately following the kicking accuracy test; thus, due to the timing of the measurement, test performance may be influenced by the players' perception of their own performance.

5. Strengths and Weaknesses

The present study is the first to investigate the effect of time-pressure on kicking accuracy, in boys, according to different times-of-day. A limitation of the current study was that dietary intake analysis was not realized before the study; however, as indicated, standardized breakfast and iso-caloric lunch were given to all boys. Another limitation of the present study was the lack of recording rectal temperature; only oral temperature was measured for ethical reasons. Furthermore, all participants were male soccer players, so our results do not generalize all populations. Finally, although we conducted an *a priori* power calculation to discern suitable statistical power, the presence of multiplicity in the statistical analyses (i.e., ANOVA) may have impacted on subsequent error rates. Nevertheless, we elected to utilize Bonferroni corrected post-hoc test, which is a conservative method of correcting for multiple testing. Notwithstanding the efforts made to ensure reliable results, the authors advocate for future studies that consider the time-of-day impact, across multiple days and bouts, to provide a more detailed understanding into the potential variability and error related to these findings.

6. Conclusions

Kicking accuracy of boys is better without time-pressure vs. with time-pressure. However, there was no-significant time-of-day effect on kicking accuracy or in perceived difficulty. Further studies are needed to explain the findings of the present study. From a practical point of view, sports scientists, clinicians, and coaches should consider the effect of time-of-day in studies, training programs, and competitive events involving boys' kicking accuracy.

Author Contributions: Conceptualization, L.M., A.G., K.T., H.C. and N.S.; methodology, L.M., A.G., K.T., H.C. and N.S.; software, L.M., A.G., C.H., K.T., O.B., H.C. and N.S.; validation, L.M., A.G., C.H., K.T., O.B., H.C., M.A.B., C.C.T.C. and N.S.; formal analysis, L.M., A.G., C.H., K.T., O.B., H.C. and N.S.; investigation, L.M., A.G. and H.C.; resources, L.M., A.G. and H.C.; data curation, L.M., A.G. and H.C.; writing—original draft preparation, L.M., A.G. and M.A.B.; writing—review and editing, L.M., A.G., C.H., K.T., O.B., H.C., M.A.B., C.C.T.C., N.S., T.R. and B.K.; visualization, L.M., A.G. and H.C.; supervision, M.A.B.; project administration, L.M., A.G. and H.C. All authors have read and agreed to the published version of the manuscript.

Funding: This research received no external funding.

Institutional Review Board Statement: The study was conducted in accordance with the Declaration of Helsinki, and the protocol was approved by the Ethics Committee (CPP SUD N° 0225/2020).

Informed Consent Statement: Informed consent was obtained from the parents//guardians of all subjects involved in the study.

Data Availability Statement: Data available on request due to privacy or ethical restrictions.

Conflicts of Interest: The authors declare no conflict of interest.

References

1. Chtourou, H.; Souissi, N. The effect of training at a specific time of day: A review. *J. Strength Cond. Res.* **2012**, *26*, 1984–2005. [CrossRef]
2. Chtourou, H.; Hammouda, O.; Souissi, H.; Chamari, K.; Chaouachi, A.; Souissi, N. Diurnal variations in physical performances related to football in adolescent soccer players. *Asian J. Sports Med.* **2012**, *3*, 139–144. [CrossRef]
3. Souissi, H.; Chtourou, H.; Chaouachi, A.; Dogui, M.; Chamari, K.; Souissi, N.; Amri, M. The effect of training at a specific time-of-day on the diurnal variations of short-term exercise performances in 10-to 11-year-old boys. *Pediatr. Exerc. Sci.* **2012**, *24*, 84–99. [CrossRef]
4. Gharbi, A.; Masmoudi, M.; Ghorbel, S.; Ben Saïd, N.; Maalej, R.; Tabka, T.; Zaouali, M. Time of Day Effect on Soccer-Specific Field Tests in Tunisian Boy Players. *Adv. Phys. Educ.* **2013**, *3*, 71–75. [CrossRef]
5. Chtourou, H.; Aloui, A.; Hammouda, O.; Souissi, H.; Chaouachi, A. Diurnal variation in long-and short-duration exercise performance and mood states in boys. *Sport Sci. Health* **2014**, *10*, 183–187. [CrossRef]
6. Reilly, T.; Atkinson, G.; Edwards, B.; Waterhouse, J.; Farrelly, K. Diurnal variation in temperature, mental and physical performance, and tasks specifically related to football (soccer). *Chronobiol. Int.* **2007**, *24*, 507–519. [CrossRef]
7. Cappaert, T.A. Time of day effect on athletic performance: An update. *J. Strength Cond. Res.* **1999**, *13*, 412–421. [CrossRef]
8. Teo, W.; Newton, M.J.; McGuigan, M.R. Circadian rhythms in exercise performance: Implications for hormonal and muscular adaptation. *J. Sports Sci. Med.* **2011**, *10*, 600–606. [PubMed]
9. Elghoul, Y.; Frikha, M.; Abdelmlak, S.; Chtourou, H.; Dammak, K.; Chamari, K.; Souissi, N. Time-of-day effect on dart-throwing performance and the perception of the difficulty of the task in 9–10 year-old boys. *Biol. Rhythm. Res.* **2014**, *4*, 523–532. [CrossRef]
10. Elghoul, Y.; Frikha, M.; Masmoudi, L.; Chtourou, L.; Chaouachi, A.; Chamari, K.; Souissi, N. Diurnal variation of cognitive performance and perceived difficulty in dart-throwing performance in 9–10 year-old boys. *Biol. Rhythm. Res.* **2014**, *5*, 789–801. [CrossRef]
11. Winget, C.M.; DeRoshia, C.W.; Holley, D.C. Circadian rhythms and athletic performance. *Med. Sci. Sports Exerc.* **1985**, *17*, 498–516. [CrossRef]
12. Masmoudi, L.; Gharbi, A.; Chtourou, H.; Souissi, N. Effect of time-of-day on soccer specific skills in children: Psychological and physiological responses. *Biol. Rhythm. Res.* **2016**, *47*, 59–68. [CrossRef]
13. Huguet, G.; Touitou, Y.; Reinberg, A. Diurnal changes in sport performance of 9- to 11-year-old school children. *Chronobiol. Int.* **1995**, *14*, 371–384. [CrossRef] [PubMed]
14. Kim, J.; Chung, S.; Tennant, L.K.; Singer, R.N.; Janelle, C.M. Minimizing error in measurement of error: A proposed method for calculation of error in a two-dimensional motor task. *Percept. Mot. Skills* **2000**, *90*, 253–261. [CrossRef] [PubMed]
15. Kubayi, A. Analysis of goal scoring patterns in the 2018 FIFA World Cup. *J. Hum. Kinet.* **2020**, *71*, 205. [CrossRef]
16. Tsaousidis, N.; Zatsiorsky, V. Two types of ball-effector interaction and their relative contribution to soccer kicking. *Hum. Mov. Sci.* **1996**, *15*, 861–876. [CrossRef]
17. Missenard, O.; Fernandez, L. Moving faster while preserving accuracy. *Neuroscience* **2011**, *197*, 233–241. [CrossRef]
18. Fitts, P.M.; Deininger, R.L. SR compatibility: Correspondence among paired elements within stimulus and response codes. *J. Exp. Psychol.* **1954**, *48*, 483. [CrossRef]
19. Van den Tillaar, R.; Ulvik, A. Influence of instruction on velocity and accuracy in soccer kicking of experienced soccer players. *J. Mot. Behav.* **2014**, *46*, 287–291. [CrossRef]
20. Frikha, M.; Derbel, M.S.; Chaâri, N.; Gharbi, A.; Chamari, K. Acute effect of stretching modalities on global coordination and kicking accuracy in 12-13 year-old soccer players. *Hum. Mov. Sci.* **2017**, *54*, 63–72. [CrossRef]
21. Reilly, T.; Farrelly, K.; Edwards, B.; Waterhouse, J. Effects of time of day on the performance of soccer-specific motor skills. In *Science and Football V*; Reilly, T., Cabri, J., Araujo, D., Eds.; Routledge: London, UK, 2004; pp. 272–274.
22. Tanner, J.M. *Growth at Adolescence*, 2nd ed.; Blackwell Science: Oxford, UK, 1962.
23. Finnoff, J.T.; Newcomer, K.; Laskowski, E.R. A valid and reliable method for measuring the kicking accuracy of soccer players. *J. Sci. Med. Sport* **2002**, *5*, 348–353. [CrossRef]
24. Foster, C.; Florhaug, J.A.; Franklin, J.; Gottschall, L.; Hrovatin, L.A.; Parker, S. A new approach to monitoring exercise training. *J. Strength Cond. Res.* **2001**, *15*, 109–115. [PubMed]
25. Hardy, C.J.; Rejeski, W.J. Not what, but how one feels: The measurement of affect during exercise. *J. Sport Exerc. Psychol.* **1989**, *11*, 304–317. [CrossRef]
26. Delignières, D.; Famose, J.P.; Thépaut-Mathieu, C.; Fleurance, P. A psychophysical study on difficulty ratings in rock climbing. *Int. J. Sports Psychol.* **1993**, *24*, 404–416.
27. McNair, D.M. Profile of mood states instrument. In *Manual for the Profile of Mood States*; Educational and Industrial Testing Service: San Diego, CA, USA, 1971; pp. 3–29.
28. Faul, F.; Erdfelder, E.; Lang, A.G.; Buchner, A. GPower 3: A flexible statistical power analysis program for the social, behavioral, and biomedical sciences. *Behav. Res. Methods* **2007**, *39*, 175–191. [CrossRef]
29. Bernard, T.; Giacomoni, M.; Gavarry, O.; Seymat, M.; Falgairette, G. Time-of-day effects in maximal anaerobic leg exercise. *Eur J. Appl. Physiol. Occup. Physiol.* **1998**, *77*, 133–138. [CrossRef] [PubMed]
30. Souissi, H.; Chaouachi, A.; Chamari, K.; Dogui, M.; Amri, M.; Souissi, N. Time-of-day effects on short-term exercise performances in 10–11-years-old Boys. *Pediatric. Exerc. Sci.* **2010**, *22*, 613–623. [CrossRef]

Article

Knee Pads Do Not Affect Physical Performance in Young Female Volleyball Players

Anja Lazić [1], Milovan Bratić [1], Stevan Stamenković [1], Slobodan Andrašić [2], Nenad Stojiljković [1] and Nebojša Trajković [1,*]

[1] Faculty of Sport and Physical Education, University of Niš, 18000 Niš, Serbia; anja.lazic96@hotmail.com (A.L.); bratic@fsfv.ni.ac.rs (M.B.); sstamenkovic.fsfv@gmail.com (S.S.); snesadif@yahoo.com (N.S.)
[2] Faculty of Economics, University of Novi Sad, 24000 Subotica, Serbia; slobodan.andrasic@ef.uns.ac.rs
* Correspondence: nele_trajce@yahoo.com; Tel.: +381-652-070-462

Abstract: Knee pads have become increasingly popular among volleyball players. Given the fact high-intensity activities that are crucial to successfully playing this sport lead to an increased risk of a knee injury, the primary use of knee pads is to prevent potential injury. However, no research has been carried out to explain the effects of knee pads on the most important physical abilities in volleyball players, thus directly affecting performance. This study was undertaken to determine the effects of knee pads on the explosive power of the lower extremities, linear speed, and agility in young female volleyball players. In two separated sessions, 84 female volleyball players (age: 14.83 ± 0.72 years; height: 163.19 ± 8.38 cm; body mass: 53.64 ± 10.42 kg; VE: 5.30 ± 3.39 years) completed squat jumps (SJ), countermovement jumps (CMJ) with and without arm swing, linear sprints at 5-m and 10-m, modified *t*-test, and 5-10-5 shuttle test. Data analyses included descriptive statistics, paired sample T-tests and use of effect size (ES). There was no statistical difference between the two conditions for SJ ($p = 0.156$; ES = 0.18), CMJ ($p = 0.817$; ES = 0.03), CMJ with arm swing ($p = 0.194$; ES = 0.14), linear sprint at 5 m ($p = 0.789$; ES = 0.03) and 10 m ($p = 0.907$; ES = −0.01), modified *t*-test ($p = 0.284$; ES = 0.13), and 5-10-5 shuttle test ($p = 0.144$; ES = 0.19). Wearing knee pads has neither an inhibitory nor positive effects on explosive power of the lower extremities, linear speed, and agility in young female volleyball players.

Keywords: jumping performance; speed; agility; team sport

1. Introduction

During a volleyball match, 80% of the points obtained are the result of high-intensity activities performed with maximal and submaximal intensity [1]. On average, volleyball players perform 250–300 high-intensity activities [2], over 100 jumps [3], and a large number of sprints up to 10 m [3], which together with technical and tactical elements [4] define volleyball as an intermittent and complex team sport, where high-intensity movements are followed by a short period of low-intensity activities [5,6]. Also, frequent changes in the rules of the game [6], the popularization and increasing in professionalism [7], specific dimensions of the court [8], and thus the high demands of the game [9], have led to a high level of physical fitness—primarily explosive power of the upper and lower extremities, speed, and agility represented as a crucial factor for successfully playing this sport at elite level [10–12]. Specifically, explosive power is manifested through a wide range of volleyball elements—ball hitting, jumps, and blocks [4,7], while speed and agility are manifested through sudden changes of movement direction [10–12], where maximal speed rarely develops [13], and movements are closely related to the unpredictable nature of actions [14]. The frequency and importance of these abilities lead to the fact that volleyball players are more prone to knee injuries, particularly to a ruptured anterior cruciate ligament [15,16]. Landings are often performed on one or both legs [17] and are associated with multiplanar cutting and pivoting movements that may increase stress load on the knee joint [14], especially in female volleyball players [18].

Prevention of potential volleyball injuries has received a lot of research attention [19]. Knee pads have become increasingly popular in volleyball players, being designed to give dynamic stability and prevent potential injury [20]. While there is no research on knee pads, knee braces have been extensively researched in rehabilitation and prevention of knee injuries in athletes [20–29]. The purpose of these braces is to effectively reduce knee valgus during lateral forces [30] without limitations in athletic performance. However, available studies addressing knee braces in injury prevention show contradictory results. While some studies have reported positive effects of knee braces in injury prevention [23,24], others have shown no effect [27–29], and Deppen with colleagues [25] together with Grace and colleagues [26], have even reported an increase in knee injury rates. Because of that, the role of knee braces is still poorly understood. This has an additional impact on athletes, who mostly avoid wearing this type of brace because of the potential negative impact on athletic performance [20,31–33]. Within this area of investigation, a number of studies [30,34–41] have reported conflicting results. Improvements in physical performance have been shown in [34,35] in contrast to those who have shown negative effects [36,40] and no effects [30,39–41] of wearing knee braces on physical performance.

However, most of these studies have utilized healthy or injured athletes, recreational athletes or non-athletes, this resulting in that the performed tests do not show the real nature of a specific competitive sport, especially in volleyball where knee pads are worn constantly and where the use of knee pads may result in decreased performance when participants become accustomed to wearing them. Since knee pads are worn by many volleyball players, it is critical to determine if wearing them significantly affects physical performance. The aim of this study was to determine the effects of knee pads on the explosive power of the lower extremities, linear speed, and agility in young female volleyball players.

2. Materials and Methods

2.1. Participants

A total of 84 young female volleyball players (age: 14.83 ± 0.72 years; height: 163.19 ± 8.38 cm; body mass: 53.64 ± 10.42 kg) volunteered to participate in the study. All participants were members of the same volleyball club. Participants had 5.30 ± 3.39 years of volleyball experience. Participants were free of injuries and medical conditions that might have placed them at risk for safe participation in the study. All participants were informed of the study procedures and provided written informed consent prior to participation, including parental consent for participants under 18 years of age.

2.2. Procedures

A repeated-measures study design was used in this study. Each participant completed two experimental trials on an indoor, hardwood volleyball court under similar environmental conditions at the same time of the day (19:00–21:00). Experimental trials were separated by 72 h. The first trial session involved testing without knee pads. After 72 h the same procedure was repeated with the use of knee pads. Before both experimental trials, participants performed a standardized warm-up, consisting of moderate-intensity jogging (5–10 min) and static and dynamic stretching (5 min) without knee pads during the first session and with knee pads during the second session. The study was conducted in accordance with the Novi Sad University Human Research Ethics Committee guidelines (ethical approval number: 20/2019; approval date of Ethic Committee approval: 20 October 2020).

2.3. Tests

2.3.1. Vertical Jump Assessment

Three tests were used to assess the explosive power of the lower extremities: squat jump (SJ), countermovement jump (CMJ), and countermovement jump with arm swing. Participants performed each jump three times. The break between each repetition of the jump was 30 s, while the break between series of new jumps was 5 min. Each participant was instructed to jump naturally and as high as they could, performing all jumps with maximal effort. The highest value of the vertical jump height for all three groups of tests was included in the statistical analysis. Optojump (Optojump, Microgate, Bolzano, Italy) was used to estimate the vertical height of the jump, and its validity and reliability were confirmed, considering low coefficients of variation (2.7%) and low random errors (+2.81 cm) [42]. The participants performed three jumps with arm swing and were instructed to jump naturally and as high as they could, performing all jumps with maximal effort.

2.3.2. Linear Speed Assessment

The linear sprinting speed was evaluated at 5 m and 10 m using a photocell system (Witty, System, Microgate, Bolzano, Italy). Each participant repeated the test three times with at least 2 min of rest between trials, and the fastest time was recorded for further statistical analysis. Photocells were placed at a distance of 5 m and 10 m from the starting line. Photocells were placed 0.4 m above the ground with an accuracy of 0.001 m/s to minimize the effect of hand swing when passing through the gate [43].

2.3.3. Agility Assessment

Agility assessment was performed using two tests—modified *t*-test and 5-10-5 shuttle test. Participants repeated each of test three times, with a break of 30 s between attempts and a 5 min break between the tests. The fastest time on agility tests was taken in further statistical analysis of the data. Modified *t*-test procedures were in accordance with Sassi et al. [44]. Upon command of the examiner, the participant sprinted towards the cone B set at the distance of 5 m and touched the base of the cone with the right hand. Then, they turned left and shuffled sideways to cone C (2.5 m), touching the base with the left hand. Then, shuffling sideways to the cone D (5 m), touching its base with the right hand, followed up by shuffle to the left to the cone B (5 m), touching its base with the left hand and running back to the cone A (5 m). The time was stopped when the start with photocell was passed by. Trials were deemed unsuccessful if participants failed to touch a designated cone, crossed their legs while shuffling, or were unable to face forward at all times. The 5-10-5 shuttle test was performed according to National Strength and Conditioning Association (NSCA) protocols [45] and measured with photo cell timing gates (Brower Timing Systems, Draper, UT). Briefly, three cones were placed five yards apart on the surface of the volleyball court. The each participant started in a three point stance and upon command sprinted right and touched the line at the first cone with his hand, the subject then turned 180 degrees and sprinted to touch the left cone line with his hand, then turned 180 degrees to sprint back to the start. The 5-10-5 shuttle run has been shown to be a reliable (ICC = 0.90, SEM = 0.12) test of change of direction [46].

2.4. Statistical Analysis

Statistical analysis was performed by the IBM SPSS statistics program (version 26.0; Inc., Chicago, IL, USA). Descriptive statistics were used to obtain basic information about the participants. The normality of data distribution was determined by Kolmogorov–Smirnov test for all dependent variables, while to determine the differences in explosive power of the lower extremities, linear speed and agility between the two conditions, the paired sample *T*-tests were used. The magnitude of difference between the two conditions was measured with effect size (ES) analyses and interpreted as: trivial ≤ 0.20; small = 0.2–0.49; moderate = 0.50–0.79; large ≥ 0.80 [47]. Data are presented as mean ± standard deviation (SD) and statistical significance level was set at $p < 0.05$

3. Results

Descriptive statistics of participants are shown in Table 1 while means and standard deviations for each dependent variable in the non-braced and braced condition are shown in Table 2. ES (effect size) comparisons between the conditions are presented in Table 2.

Table 1. Descriptive statistics of participants.

Outcome Measure (Unit)	N	Min	Max	Mean ± SD
Age (year)	84	12	20	14.83 ± 0.72
VE (year)	84	1	15	5.30 ± 3.39
Height (cm)	84	147.0	179.5	163.19 ± 8.38
Body mass (kg)	84	35.0	85.7	53.64 ± 10.42

VE—volleyball experience; N—a total number of participants; SD—standard deviation.

Table 2. Differences and effect size values between the conditions.

Outcome Measure	Condition		p Value	ES
	Without Knee Pads	With Knee Pads		
Vertical jump height				
SJ (cm)	23.55 ± 5.03	24.47 ± 5.06	0.156	0.18—trivial
CMJ without arm swing (cm)	24.46 ± 5.46	24.61 ± 5.56	0.817	0.03—trivial
CMJ with arm swing (cm)	29.91 ± 6.40	30.90 ± 7.30	0.194	0.14—trivial
Linear sprint speed				
5 m—sprint (s)	1.25 ± 0.15	1.25 ± 0.12	0.789	0.03—trivial
10 m—sprint (s)	2.18 ± 0.18	2.17 ± 0.17	0.907	−0.01—trivial
Agility				
modified t-test (s)	7.40 ± 0.58	7.48 ± 0.64	0.284	0.13—trivial
5-10-5 test (s)	5.96 ± 0.35	6.03 ± 0.40	0.144	0.19—trivial

SJ—squat jump; CMJ—counter movement jump; p value—significant difference, $p = 0.05$; ES—effect size.

Table 1 shows that the mean age of the 84 female volleyball players was 14.83 ± 0.72 years (range: 12–20 years), with a mean height of 163.19 ± 8.38 cm (range: 147.0–179.5 cm) and mean weight 53.64 ± 10.42 kg (range: 35.0–85.7 kg); mean volleyball experience was 5.30 ± 3.39 years (range: 1–15 years).

The Kolmogorov–Smirnov tests showed that data were normally distributed and homogeneity of variance was confirmed using the Levene's test. Paired sample T-tests were used to determine potential differences between braced and non-braced conditions in height of vertical jumping, linear sprinting speed, and agility. Table 2 shows non-significant differences found for any variable between the two conditions. Wearing knee pads resulted in a trivial, non-significant increase in SJ (ES = 0.18), CMJ (ES = 0.03) and non-significant increase in CMJ with arm swing (ES = 0.14); trivial, non-significant reduction in the time required to perform linear sprint at 5 m (ES = 0.03); and trivial, non-significant reduction in the time required to perform linear sprint at 10 m (ES = −0.01). Finally, wearing knee pads resulted in trivial, non-significant increase in the time required to perform modified t-test (ES = 0.13) and 5-10-5 shuttle test (ES = 0.19).

4. Discussion

The aim of this study was to determine the effects of wearing knee pads on young female volleyball players, on the explosive power of the lower extremities, linear speed, and agility. The results showed that there were no statistically significant differences between the two conditions and that wearing knee pads did not improve, but also did not inhibit specific volleyball performance.

Although a considerable body of research has been done on the effects of knee bracing in injured athletes [35,48,49] and non-athletes [30,39], less attention has been paid to the population of interest [41,50,51]. Past studies in non-injured populations have yielded some important insights into the effects of wearing a knee brace on height during vertical jumping [30,39,41,50,51]. Taken altogether, the data presented here provide evidence that the braces do not affect vertical jump height. Studies of Batlaci et al. [30] and Veldhuizen et al. [39] investigated vertical jump height in young, uninjured participants and found no statistically significant differences between braced and non – braced conditions. However, due to the sample of participants [30,39] as well as the selection of the tests for assessing the explosive power of the lower extremities [30], these findings do not aplly to athletes. Substantially, studies involving athletes [41,50] have not defined definite differences between the two conditions. Rishiraj and colleagues [50] conducted five testing sessions in each condition. Statistically significant differences were noticeable at the initial testing session, but at the final testing session, no difference was found in the vertical jump. Mortaza and colleagues [41] included 31 male athletes in one testing session and found no effect of bracing on vertical jump. While we could not find initial significant effects of bracing in volleyball players, in braced and non-braced condition, Rishiraj et al. [50] and Veldhuizen et al. [39] found initial, acute decrease in vertical jump height. A possible explanation could be given by Aktas and Baltaci [51], who emphasize that the external load exerted by the knee braces can apply excessive pressure to the skin and change the physiology by inhibiting the mechanoreceptors of the knee, which may results in negative acute effects of knee bracing. However, there is no reliable evidence that this decrease is due to wearing knee braces, given that after the period of 14 h [50] and 28 days [39], there were no statistically significant differences between braced and non—braced conditions. Also, in this study, the period between the trials was 72 h, it should be added that volleyball players use knee pads more and longer than other athletes, so we should not rule out potential earlier adaptation to wearing a pad as a mediator of non—significant differences.

In contrast to the findings of this study, where sprint performance at 5 m and 10 m did not differ between braced and non-braced conditions, previous studies [39,50,52–54] have demonstrated that knee braces inhibit running velocity at short distances. These findings are less surprising if we consider the sample of participants. Veldhuzen et al. [39] included eight healthy volunteers and found that sprinting time during 60 m Dash test was 4% longer than in non-braced volunteers. Similarly, Rishiraj et al. [50] reported longer time at 10 m sprint. However, both studies concluded that after getting accustomed to knee brace, after 4 weeks [39] and 14 h [50], results came back to baseline compared to unbraced condition. In other studies, participants were rugby players [52], young male athletes [50], and young college athletes in unspecified sports [53]. These findings are not generalizable to volleyball players. A possible reason for this discrepancy might be that sprint performance depends on the type of knee brace. In a study conducted by Green and colleagues [55], the effects of six different knee braces on speed and agility were analyzed. Four out of six braces negatively affected athletic performane. This finding is congruent with the work of Albright et al. [54], which showed that longer time required to complete sprint tests depends on a variety of factors, among which the most important are the weight and design of the knee brace. The weight of the knee brace leads to altered activity of the knee extensors and hip flexors [53], which are the most active muscles while jogging, running or sprinting [56]. However, a more relevant study to explain the results obtained is a study of Stephens [57] who reported that knee bracing had no effect on sprint speed. This is a statement with a strong background, because basketball and volleyball have many more similarities as team, indoor sports with a specific manifestation of physical fitness [58] than other sports presented in the disscusion.

Wearing a knee brace may negatively affect agility and athletic performance [59], taking into account the fact that agility is a crucial ability in many sports. However, there was no statistical difference between the two conditions in time required to complete the agility tests with or without knee pads. A limited number of studies [55,59,60] have addressed the fact that agility maneuvers are not affected by knee bracing. However, while the former study of Rishiraj et al. [60] showed no differences between the two conditions in agility slalom test and the figure-of-eight test, the latter study, which included 27 young male athletes [50], resulted in initially longer time required to complete agility test in braced-group, but after 14 h, results came back to baseline as in unbraced condition. They attributed decrease in performance to the adaptation to wearing a knee brace. The weakness of this research is that they examined agility without cutting movements, in regard to a straight line. Similarly, Green et al. [55] showed that agility performance depends on the type of knee brace, where significant differences were found only with one of six braces.

These findings are less surprising if we consider that the volleyball players were well-rested during the assessment, without the previous high-intensity activities, so it would be more relevant to determine the impact of knee pads on vertical jump, speed, and agility in condition of acute fatigue, similar to that during a volleyball match. A possible reason for this discrepancy might be that non-significant differences are probably a consequence of the weight and design of volleyball knee pads, which are lighter, with different designs, in relation to the majority of knee braces presented in the discussion. At present our dataset is limited to studies which do not address knee pads or a specific volleyball population. Therefore, these findings are not sufficient to determine whether knee pads inhibit or improve volleyball performance. Future studies are to be carried out to explore effects of specific knee pads in volleyball players, taking into account their wide use in volleyball.

5. Conclusions

Pointing to the majority of volleyball players who use knee pads, this research was conducted with the aim of determining the effect of knee pads on important factors of volleyball performance. The conclusion is that wearing knee pads has neither an inhibitory nor a positive effect on the explosive power of the lower extremities; linear speed; and agility in young female volleyball players. However, to our knowledge, this is the first study that tried to examine the effects of knee pads in athletes and the first study that involved a specific population of volleyball players. Considering the importance of high level of these abilities for successful volleyball performance and at the same time the wide use of knee pads in volleyball players, further research in this area of is needed. This study provides data that will help coaches and volleyball players in resolving doubts about the use of knee pads for players of all ages, especially for young players whose locomotor system has not yet been formed. The findings of this study highlight that wearing knee pads do not deteriorate the physical performance of volleyball players and that their further use is desirable for the primary purpose, which is the prevention of potential knee injuries and consequences of frequent falls, which all together may have a positive impact on the psychological status and overall performance of the athlete. Moreover this study supports researchers who will try to examine and explain the impact of knee pads and to what extent they affect the prevention of potential knee injuries in volleyball players.

Author Contributions: Conceptualization, N.T., N.S. and M.B.; methodology, N.S.; software, S.A. and M.B.; validation, S.S., S.A. and N.S.; formal analysis, S.S., and M.B.; investigation, A.L.; resources, A.L.; data curation, S.A.; writing—original draft preparation, N.T.; writing—review and editing, A.L.; visualization, A.L.; supervision, N.T. All authors have read and agreed to the published version of the manuscript.

Funding: This research was funded by the Serbian Ministry of Education, Science and Technological Development.

Institutional Review Board Statement: The study was conducted according to the guidelines of the Declaration of Helsinki, and approved by the Novi Sad University Human Research Ethics Committee guidelines (ethical approval number: 20/2019).

Informed Consent Statement: Informed consent was obtained from all subjects involved in the study.

Conflicts of Interest: The authors declare no conflict of interest.

References

1. Voigt, H.; Vetter, K. The value of strength-diagnostic for the structure of jump training in volleyball. *Eur. J. Sport Sci.* **2003**, *3*, 1–10. [CrossRef]
2. Hasegawa, H.; Dziados, J.; Newton, R.U.; Fry, A.C.; Kraemer, W.J.; Häkkinen, K. Periodized training programmes for athletes. In *Handbook of Sports Medicine and Science: Strength Training for Sport*; Wiley Blackwell: Hoboken, NJ, USA, 2008.
3. Jastrzebski, Z.; Wnorowski, K.; Mikolajewski, R.; Jaskulska, E.; Radziminski, L.; Activity, P. The effect of a 6-week plyometric training on explosive power in volleyball players. *Balt. J. Health Phys. Act.* **2014**, *6*, 79. [CrossRef]

4. Marques, M.C.; Van Den Tillaar, R.; Vescovi, J.D.; González-Badillo, J.; Research, C. Changes in strength and power performance in elite senior female professional volleyball players during the in-season: A case study. *J. Strength Cond. Res.* **2008**, *22*, 1147–1155. [CrossRef] [PubMed]
5. Gabbett, T.; Georgieff, B.; Research, C. Physiological and anthropometric characteristics of Australian junior national, state, and novice volleyball players. *J. Strength Cond. Res.* **2007**, *21*, 902–908. [PubMed]
6. Sheppard, J.M.; Gabbett, T.J.; Stanganelli, L.-C.R.; Research, C. An analysis of playing positions in elite men's volleyball: Considerations for competition demands and physiologic characteristics. *J. Strength Cond. Res.* **2009**, *23*, 1858–1866. [CrossRef] [PubMed]
7. Marques, M.; González-Badillo, J.; Kluka, D.; Journal, C. In-season strength training male professional volleyball athletes. *Strength Cond. J.* **2006**, *28*, 2–12.
8. Grgantov, Z.; Milić, M.; Katić, R. Identification af explosive power factors as predictors of player quality in young female volleyball players. *Coll. Antropol.* **2013**, *37*, 61–68.
9. Skazalski, C.; Whiteley, R.; Bahr, R. High jump demands in professional volleyball—Large variability exists between players and player positions. *Scand. J. Med. Sci. Sports* **2018**, *28*, 2293–2298. [CrossRef]
10. Kim, Y.-Y.; Park, S.-E. Comparison of whole-body vibration exercise and plyometric exercise to improve isokinetic muscular strength, jumping performance and balance of female volleyball players. *J. Phys. Ther. Sci.* **2016**, *28*, 3140–3144. [CrossRef]
11. Trajković, N.; Krističević, T.; Baić, M. Effects of plyometric training on sport-specific tests in female volleyball players. *Age* **2016**, *17*, 20–24.
12. Lidor, R.; Ziv, G.; Research, C. Physical and physiological attributes of female volleyball players—A review. *J. Strength Cond. Res.* **2010**, *24*, 1963–1973. [CrossRef]
13. Johnson, T.M.; Brown, L.E.; Coburn, J.W.; Judelson, D.A.; Khamoui, A.V.; Tran, T.T.; Uribe, B.P.; Research, C. Effect of four different starting stances on sprint time in collegiate volleyball players. *J. Strength Cond. Res.* **2010**, *24*, 2641–2646. [CrossRef]
14. Zahradnik, D.; Jandacka, D.; Farana, R.; Uchytil, J.; Hamill, J. Identification of types of landings after blocking in volleyball associated with risk of ACL injury. *Eur. J. Sport Sci.* **2017**, *17*, 241–248. [CrossRef] [PubMed]
15. Lobietti, R.; Coleman, S.; Pizzichillo, E.; Merni, F. Landing techniques in volleyball. *J. Sports Sci.* **2010**, *28*, 1469–1476. [CrossRef]
16. Leporace, G.; Praxedes, J.; Pereira, G.R.; Pinto, S.M.; Chagas, D.; Metsavaht, L.; Chame, F.; Batista, L.A. Influence of a preventive training program on lower limb kinematics and vertical jump height of male volleyball athletes. *Phys. Ther. Sport* **2013**, *14*, 35–43. [CrossRef] [PubMed]
17. Tillman, M.D.; Hass, C.J.; Brunt, D.; Bennett, G. Jumping and landing techniques in elite women's volleyball. *J. Sports Sci. Med.* **2004**, *3*, 30. [PubMed]
18. Hughes, G.; Watkins, J.; Owen, N. The effects of opposition and gender on knee kinematics and ground reaction force during landing from volleyball block jumps. *Res. Q. Exerc. Sport* **2010**, *81*, 384–391. [CrossRef]
19. Gouttebarge, V.; van Sluis, M.; Verhagen, E.; Zwerver, J. The prevention of musculoskeletal injuries in volleyball: The systematic development of an intervention and its feasibility. *Inj. Epidemiol.* **2017**, *4*, 25. [CrossRef]
20. Rishiraj, N.; Taunton, J.E.; Lloyd-Smith, R.; Woollard, R.; Regan, W.; Clement, D.B. The potential role of prophylactic/functional knee bracing in preventing knee ligament injury. *Sports Med.* **2009**, *39*, 937–960. [CrossRef]
21. Pietrosimone, B.G.; Grindstaff, T.L.; Linens, S.W.; Uczekaj, E.; Hertel, J. A systematic review of prophylactic braces in the prevention of knee ligament injuries in collegiate football players. *J. Athl. Train.* **2008**, *43*, 409–415. [CrossRef]
22. Sitler, M.; Ryan, C.J.; Hopkinson, L.W.; Wheeler, L.J.; Santomier, J.; Kolb, L.R.; Polley, C.D. The efficacy of a prophylactic knee brace to reduce knee injuries in football: A prospective, randomized study at West Point. *Am. J. Sports Med.* **1990**, *18*, 310–315. [CrossRef]
23. Van Tiggelen, D.; Witvrouw, E.; Roget, P.; Cambier, D.; Danneels, L.; Verdonk, R. Effect of bracing on the prevention of anterior knee pain—A prospective randomized study. *Knee Surg. Sports Traumatol. Arthrosc.* **2004**, *12*, 434–439. [CrossRef]
24. Fleming, B.C.; Renstrom, P.A.; Beynnon, B.D.; Engstrom, B.; Peura, G. The influence of functional knee bracing on the anterior cruciate ligament strain biomechanics in weightbearing and nonweightbearing knees. *Am. J. Sports Med.* **2000**, *28*, 815–824. [CrossRef]
25. Deppen, R.J.; Landfried, M.; Therapy, S.P. Efficacy of prophylactic knee bracing in high school football players. *J. Orthop. Sports Phys. Ther.* **1994**, *20*, 243–246. [CrossRef] [PubMed]
26. Grace, T.G.; Skipper, B.; Newberry, J.; Nelson, M.; Sweetser, E.; Rothman, M.L. Prophylactic knee braces and injury to the lower extremity. *J. Bone Jt. Surg.* **1988**, *70*, 422–427. [CrossRef]
27. Risberg, M.; Beynnon, B.; Peura, G.; Uh, B.S. Proprioception after anterior cruciate ligament reconstruction with and without bracing. *Knee Surg. Sports Traumatol. Arthrosc.* **1999**, *7*, 303–309. [CrossRef]
28. Rovere, G.D.; Clarke, T.J.; Yates, C.S.; Burley, K. Retrospective comparison of taping and ankle stabilizers in preventing ankle injuries. *Am. J. Sports Med.* **1988**, *16*, 228–233. [CrossRef]
29. Rovere, G.D.; Haupt, H.A.; Yates, C.S. Prophylactic knee bracing in college football. *Am. J. Sports Med.* **1987**, *15*, 111–116. [CrossRef]
30. Baltaci, G.; Aktas, G.; Camci, E.; Oksuz, S.; Yildiz, S.; Kalaycioglu, T. The effect of prophylactic knee bracing on performance: Balance, proprioception, coordination, and muscular power. *Knee Surg. Sports Traumatol. Arthrosc.* **2011**, *19*, 1722–1728. [CrossRef] [PubMed]

31. McDevitt, E.R.; Taylor, D.C.; Miller, M.D.; Gerber, J.P.; Ziemke, G.; Hinkin, D.; Uhorchak, J.M.; Arciero, R.A.; St. Pierre, P. Functional bracing after anterior cruciate ligament reconstruction: A prospective, randomized, multicenter study. *Am. J. Sports Med.* **2004**, *32*, 1887–1892. [CrossRef]
32. Najibi, S.; Albright, J.P. The use of knee braces, part 1: Prophylactic knee braces in contact sports. *Am. J. Sports Med.* **2005**, *33*, 602–611. [CrossRef]
33. Risberg, M.A.; Holm, I.; Steen, H.; Eriksson, J.; Ekeland, A. The effect of knee bracing after anterior cruciate ligament reconstruction. *Am. J. Sports Med.* **1999**, *27*, 76–83. [CrossRef]
34. Cook, F.F.; Tibone, J.E.; Redfern, F.C. A dynamic analysis of a functional brace for anterior cruciate ligament insufficiency. *Am. J. Sports Med.* **1989**, *17*, 519–524. [CrossRef]
35. Rebel, M.; Paessler, H. The effect of knee brace on coordination and neuronal leg muscle control: An early postoperative functional study in anterior cruciate ligament reconstructed patients. *Knee Surg. Sports Traumatol. Arthrosc.* **2001**, *9*, 272–281. [CrossRef]
36. Wu, G.K.; Ng, G.Y.; Mak, A.F. Effects of knee bracing on the functional performance of patients with anterior cruciate ligament reconstruction. *Arch. Phys. Med. Rehabil.* **2001**, *82*, 282–285. [CrossRef]
37. Mortaza, N.; Osman, N.A.; Jamshidi, A.A.; Razjouyan, J. Influence of functional knee bracing on the isokinetic and functional tests of anterior cruciate ligament deficient patients. *PLoS ONE* **2013**, *8*, e64308. [CrossRef] [PubMed]
38. Tegner, Y.; Lysholm, J.; Surgery, R. Derotation brace and knee function in patients with anterior cruciate ligament tears. *Arthrosc. J. Arthrosc. Relat. Surg.* **1985**, *1*, 264–267. [CrossRef]
39. Veldhuizen, J.; Koene, F.; Oostvogel, H.; Thiel, T.P.H.; Verstappen, F.J.I. The effects of a supportive knee brace on leg performance in healthy subjects. *Int. J. Sports Med.* **1991**, *12*, 577–580. [CrossRef] [PubMed]
40. Sforzo, G.A.; Chen, N.; Gold, C.A.; Frye, P.A. The effect of prophylactic knee bracing on performance. *Med. Sci. Sports Exerc.* **1989**, *21*, 254–257. [CrossRef]
41. Mortaza, N.; Ebrahimi, I.; Jamshidi, A.A.; Abdollah, V.; Kamali, M.; Abas, W.A.B.W.; Abu Osman, N.A. The effects of a prophylactic knee brace and two neoprene knee sleeves on the performance of healthy athletes: A crossover randomized controlled trial. *PLoS ONE* **2012**, *7*, e50110. [CrossRef] [PubMed]
42. Glatthorn, J.F.; Gouge, S.; Nussbaumer, S.; Stauffacher, S.; Impellizzeri, F.M.; Maffiuletti, N.A. Validity and reliability of Optojump photoelectric cells for estimating vertical jump height. *J. Strength Cond. Res.* **2011**, *25*, 556–560. [CrossRef]
43. Yeadon, M.; Kato, T.; Kerwin, D. Measuring running speed using photocells. *J. Sports Sci.* **1999**, *17*, 249–257. [CrossRef]
44. Sassi, R.H.; Dardouri, W.; Yahmed, M.H.; Gmada, N.; Mahfoudhi, M.E.; Gharbi, Z. Relative and absolute reliability of a modified agility T-test and its relationship with vertical jump and straight sprint. *J. Strength Cond. Res.* **2009**, *23*, 1644–1651. [CrossRef]
45. Triplett, N. *Speed and Agility*; Human Kinetics: Champaign, IL, USA, 2012; pp. 253–274.
46. Stewart, P.F.; Turner, A.N.; Miller, S.C. Reliability, factorial validity, and interrelationships of five commonly used change of direction speed tests. *Scand. J. Med. Sci. Sports* **2014**, *24*, 500–506. [CrossRef]
47. Cohen, J. *Statistical Power Analysis for the Behavioral Sciences*; Academic Press: Cambridge, MA, USA, 2013.
48. Dickerson, L.C.; Peebles, A.T.; Moskal, J.T.; Miller, T.K.; Queen, R.M. Physical performance improves with time and a functional knee brace in Athletes after ACL reconstruction. *Orthop. J. Sports Med.* **2020**, *8*, 8. [CrossRef] [PubMed]
49. Moon, J.; Kim, H.; Lee, J.; Panday, S.B. Effect of wearing a knee brace or sleeve on the knee joint and anterior cruciate ligament force during drop jumps: A clinical intervention study. *Knee* **2018**, *25*, 1009–1015. [CrossRef] [PubMed]
50. Rishiraj, N.; Taunton, J.E.; Lloyd-Smith, R.; Regan, W.; Niven, B.; Woollard, R. Effect of functional knee brace use on acceleration, agility, leg power and speed performance in healthy athletes. *Br. J. Sports Med.* **2011**, *45*, 1230–1237. [CrossRef] [PubMed]
51. Aktas, G.; Baltaci, G. Does kinesiotaping increase knee muscles strength and functional performance? *Isokinet. Exerc. Sci.* **2011**, *19*, 149–155. [CrossRef]
52. Kruger, T.H.; Coetsee, M.F.; Davies, S.E. The effect of Prophylactic knee bracing on selected performance patameters. *Afr. J. Phys. Act. Health Sci.* **2003**, *9*, 40–57. [CrossRef]
53. Borsa, P.A.; Lephart, S.M.; Fu, F.H. Muscular and functional performance characteristics of individuals wearing prophylactic knee braces. *J. Athl. Train.* **1993**, *28*, 336.
54. Albright, J.P.; Saterbak, A.; Stokes, J. Use of knee braces in sport. *Sports Med.* **1995**, *20*, 281–301. [CrossRef]
55. Greene, D.L.; Hamson, K.R.; Bay, R.C.; Bryce, C.D. Effects of protective knee bracing on speed and agility. *Am. J. Sports Med.* **2000**, *28*, 453–459. [CrossRef] [PubMed]
56. Mann, R.A.; Moran, G.T.; Dougherty, S.E. Comparative electromyography of the lower extremity in jogging, running, and sprinting. *Am. J. Sports Med.* **1986**, *14*, 501–510. [CrossRef]
57. Stephens, D.L. The effects of functional knee braces on speed in collegiate basketball players. *J. Orthop. Sports Phys. Ther.* **1995**, *22*, 259–262. [CrossRef] [PubMed]
58. Peña, J.; Moreno-Doutres, D.; Coma, J.; Cook, M.; Buscà, B. Anthropometric and fitness profile of high-level basketball, handball and volleyball players. *Rev. Andal. Med. Deport.* **2018**, *11*, 30–35. [CrossRef]
59. Bodendorfer, B.M.; Arnold, N.R.; Shu, H.T.; Leary, E.V.; Cook, J.L.; Gray, A.D.; Guess, T.M.; Sherman, S.L. Do neoprene sleeves and prophylactic knee braces affect neuromuscular control and cutting agility? *Phys. Ther. Sport* **2019**, *39*, 23–31. [CrossRef]
60. Rishiraj, N.; Taunton, J.; Clement, D.; Lloyd-Smith, R.; Regan, W.; Woollard, R. The role of functional knee bracing in a dynamic setting. *N. Z. J. Sports Med.* **2000**, *28*, 54–61. [CrossRef]

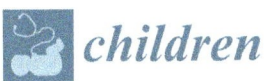

Article

Foundational Movement Skills and Play Behaviors during Recess among Preschool Children: A Compositional Analysis

Lawrence Foweather [1,*], Matteo Crotti [1], Jonathan D. Foulkes [1], Mareesa V. O'Dwyer [1], Till Utesch [2], Zoe R. Knowles [1], Stuart J. Fairclough [3], Nicola D. Ridgers [4] and Gareth Stratton [5]

[1] Research Institute for Sport & Exercise Sciences, Liverpool John Moores University, Liverpool L3 3AT, UK; M.Crotti@2016.ljmu.ac.uk (M.C.); J.D.Foulkes@ljmu.ac.uk (J.D.F.); modwyer@earlychildhoodireland.ie (M.V.O.); Z.R.Knowles@ljmu.ac.uk (Z.R.K.)
[2] Institute of Educational Sciences, University of Münster, 48149 Münster, Germany; till.utesch@uni-muenster.de
[3] Department of Sport and Physical Activity, Edge Hill University, Ormskirk L39 4QP, UK; faircls@edgehill.ac.uk
[4] Institute for Physical Activity and Nutrition, School of Exercise and Nutrition Sciences, Deakin University, Geelong 3220, Australia; nicky.ridgers@deakin.edu.au
[5] College of Engineering, Swansea University, Swansea SA2 8PP, UK; G.Stratton@swansea.ac.uk
* Correspondence: L.Foweather@ljmu.ac.uk

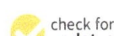

Citation: Foweather, L.; Crotti, M.; Foulkes, J.D.; O'Dwyer, M.V.; Utesch, T.; Knowles, Z.R.; Fairclough, S.J.; Ridgers, N.D.; Stratton, G. Foundational Movement Skills and Play Behaviors during Preschool Children: A Compositional Analysis. Children 2021, 8, 543. https://doi.org/10.3390/children8070543

Academic Editor: Rhodri S. Lloyd

Received: 31 May 2021
Accepted: 23 June 2021
Published: 24 June 2021

Publisher's Note: MDPI stays neutral with regard to jurisdictional claims in published maps and institutional affiliations.

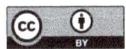

Copyright: © 2021 by the authors. Licensee MDPI, Basel, Switzerland. This article is an open access article distributed under the terms and conditions of the Creative Commons Attribution (CC BY) license (https://creativecommons.org/licenses/by/4.0/).

Abstract: This study aimed to examine the associations between play behaviors during preschool recess and foundational movement skills (FMS) in typically developing preschool children. One hundred and thirty-three children (55% male; mean age 4.7 ± 0.5 years) from twelve preschools were video-assessed for six locomotor and six object-control FMS using the Champs Motor Skill Protocol. A modified System for Observing Children's Activity and Relationships during Play assessed play behaviors during preschool recess. Associations between the composition of recess play behaviors with FMS were analyzed using compositional data analysis and linear regression. Results: Relative to time spent in other types of play behaviors, time spent in play without equipment was positively associated with total and locomotor skills, while time spent in locomotion activities was negatively associated with total and locomotor skills. No associations were found between activity level and group size play behavior compositions and FMS. The findings suggest that activity type play behaviors during recess are associated with FMS. While active games without equipment appear beneficial, preschool children may need a richer playground environment, including varied fixed and portable equipment, to augment the play-based development of FMS.

Keywords: motor skills; fundamental movement skills; play; preschool; early childhood education centers; physical literacy; young children; early childhood; cross-sectional; observational

1. Introduction

Early childhood is recognized as a critical period for the development of foundational movement skills (FMS) [1–3]. FMS is a relatively new term that includes both traditionally conceptualized *fundamental* movement skills such as stability (e.g., sitting, standing, balancing on a foot), locomotor (e.g., running, jumping, crawling), and object control (e.g., striking, catching, throwing) skills, as well as other skills that support lifelong engagement in physical activity (e.g., squatting, cycling, swimming) [1]. 'Foundational' refers to these skills providing an 'underlying base or support', with the development of greater competency in many skills providing more options for physical activity across the life course [1]. FMS are typically poorly developed in preschool children as they find themselves at the rudimentary stage of development [4,5]. Young children will not acquire proficiency in FMS through growth and maturation alone: the rate and extent of FMS development is dependent on the interplay between environmental (e.g., access to equipment) and individual (e.g., confidence) factors [6–8] and is therefore non-linear and idiosyncratic [9].

Developing proficiency in these skills through childhood is important, as FMS provide an underlying base or support for successful participation in physical activities and sport across the life course [1,7,10–12]. For example, preschool children with higher FMS competence are more likely to have higher physical fitness and physical activity levels later in life [13,14]. Furthermore, accumulative evidence highlights the beneficial effects of FMS competence on wider aspects of child development. FMS have been linked to key elements of school readiness [15], including cognitive [16,17], language [18], and social [19] outcomes. Moreover, FMS level has been found to be inversely related with body mass index (BMI) [20,21] and positively associated with physical activity behaviors in preschool children [22–24].

Play is suggested to be an important context for FMS in the early years [9,25–28] and is characterized by activities that are freely chosen, self-directed, intrinsically motivated, and free from many constraints of objective reality [29–31]. The proportion of time spent in unstructured play reaches its peak in the preschool period before declining rapidly in the primary school years [31]. Through play, young children have opportunities to explore their environment and develop and practice FMS [9,25–27]. Play has also been noted for its potential to foster children's strength, endurance, cognition, and prosocial behaviors, which in turn could mediate FMS development [28,31–35]. Active play [36], risky play [37], and outdoor play [38,39] are considered particularly beneficial for young children's physical development, challenging their movement abilities such as balance, agility, coordination, and spatial awareness, as well as nurturing physical activity behaviors through activities that conjure up feelings of thrill and excitement. Despite these assertions, empirical studies examining the associations between FMS competence and play behaviors are lacking [40,41]. Indeed, studies to date have focused on environmental factors such as playground size rather than what play behaviors children are engaged in within play settings and with whom [40,41]. Such evidence could be used to identify what play behaviors could be targeted in FMS interventions for preschoolers.

An important context where many young children spend a significant proportion of their time is at preschool (i.e., early education and childcare settings such as kindergartens, nurseries, day care centers, and preschools—both public and private). In Western Europe and including the United Kingdom, over 90% of three-to-five-year-old children are enrolled at preschool [42]. In England, all three- and four-year-old children receive 15 h of free preschool education for 38 weeks of the year. English educational settings follow the Early Years Foundation Stage curriculum [43], which has emphasised play-based learning and development in several core areas including physical development, personal, social, and emotional development, and communication and language, among others. At preschool, young children can foster physical development through unstructured and outdoor free play during several regularly scheduled break times each day (recess periods). Increased levels of moderate-to-vigorous intensity physical activity within recess periods indicates that this may be an important environment for play and FMS development in a preschooler's day [44]. A small positive relationship between children's overall FMS competence and the playground size in the preschool setting has also been noted [45]. Whilst this latter study examined several preschool environmental characteristics, to the best of our knowledge, no study has examined the relationship between FMS and young children's play behaviors during preschool recess.

The aim of the present study, therefore, was to examine the associations between play behaviors and FMS in typically developing preschool children during recess at preschool. Play behaviors during recess occur in a finite time window and are therefore mutually exclusive and co-dependent on each other (i.e., time spent in one behavior can only be changed by increasing or reducing time spent in at least one of the other play behaviors by the same duration). Thus, play behaviors should be analyzed and interpreted relative to one another as opposed to in isolation [46,47]. The present study therefore used compositional data analysis (CoDA) as a statistical approach for the inferential analysis of recess play behavior data against FMS outcomes [46,47]. CoDA is increasingly used in the field and robust to issues such as collinearity [47]. To our knowledge, this is the first study to use CoDA to analyze the association between recess play behaviors and FMS.

2. Methods

2.1. Design

This research was part of the Active Play project, which is described in detail elsewhere [44] and was approved by the University Ethics Committee (ref. 09/SPS/027). In summary, Active Play consisted of a 6-week educational programme conducted during class time that involved staff and children from preschools within disadvantaged communities and targeted children's physical activity levels, FMS, fitness, and self-confidence. The data used in this cross-sectional study were collected through two phases of baseline assessments conducted during October 2009 and March 2010 to maximize recruitment and control for the influence of seasonal effects.

2.2. Settings and Participants

Twelve preschools situated in a large urban city in Northwest England and located within neighborhoods within the highest 10% for national deprivation [48] were randomly selected and invited to participate in the study. All of the preschools provided informed gatekeeper consent to participate. All children aged three- to- five-years-old at the study preschools were invited to participate and were required to return informed written parental consent, demographic information (home postcode, the child's ethnicity and date of birth, and the mother's highest level of education) and medical assessment forms. From the 673 eligible children, parental consent was obtained for 240 children (35% response rate). No children had any known medical conditions that could affect motor proficiency or participation in physical activity.

2.3. Measures

2.3.1. Foundational Movement Skills

The Children's Activity and Movement Assessment Study (CHAMPS) Motor Skill Protocol (CMSP) was used to assess the preschoolers' FMS [49]. CMSP is a valid and reliable tool developed for three-to-five-year-old children and assesses process characteristics in six locomotor (run, broad jump, leap, hop, gallop, and slide) and six object-control (overarm throw, stationary strike, kick, catch, underhand roll, and stationary dribble) skills [49]. Following a single demonstration of each skill by a trained research assistant, children performed two trials of each skill in a standardized order while working in small groups of 2–4 children. Trials took place at preschool within either indoor halls or on outdoor playgrounds, depending on available facilities, and were recorded using a tripod-mounted video camera for later analysis. Skill components were subsequently marked as present (scored 1) or absent (scored 0) against the process criteria (e.g., arms extend forwards and upwards in the horizontal jump) by a single trained assessor [49]. Inter-rater reliability with an experienced assessor was established prior to assessment using pre-coded videotapes of 10 children, with 83.9% agreement across the twelve FMS (range 72.9–89.3%). The total number of skill components checked as present over two trials was summed to give a composite total skill score (possible range: 0–142 skill components), whilst locomotor (0–64 skill components) and object-control (0–78 skill components) subtest scores were created by summing the scores of skills within each subscale.

2.3.2. Play Behaviors

A modified version of the System for Observing Children's Activity and Relationships during Play (SOCARP) was used to assess preschool children's play behaviors [50]. SOCARP is a validated tool designed to simultaneously assess multiple aspects of play using time sampling techniques where a 10 s observation period is followed by a 10 s recording period [50]. SOCARP codes play behaviors in four categories: *activity level* (lying, sitting, standing, walking, and very active), *group size* (alone, small group of 2–4 individuals, medium group of 5–9 individuals, and large group of ≥10 individuals), *activity type* (sport (e.g., football, tennis]), active games (e.g., dancing, throwing, and catching), sedentary (e.g., reading, artwork) and locomotion (e.g., running/walking/jogging/skipping that is not part of an active game, such as transitioning from one activity to another), and *interactions* (no interaction, physical sportsmanship, verbal sportsmanship, physical conflict, verbal conflict, and ignore). For this study, SOCARP was modified to enable a more detailed examination of play behaviors of young children. Specifically, the 'sport' category was removed from the *activity type* variable and the 'active games' category was divided into two categories: 'active games with equipment' (fixed (e.g., climbing frame) or portable/loose parts (e.g., balls or socio-dramatic props such as teacups)) or 'active games without equipment' (e.g., chasing games/rough and tumble). Furthermore, the 'sedentary' *activity type* category was divided into 'sedentary' (i.e., non-play sedentary behaviors, e.g., viewing others' games but sitting as a spectator) and 'quiet play' (i.e., play-based sedentary behaviors, e.g., sitting playing board games). Each child was filmed for 5 min by a research assistant during a single morning (~20 min), lunch (~45 min), or afternoon (~20 min) recess period, which took place outdoors on the preschool play area. For each 10 s recording period, play behaviors across each category were coded, and the number of intervals (units) per behavior category were summed for use in the statistical analysis. A trained observer (MOD) retrospectively coded the play behaviors using video recordings. Observer training was conducted through coding a prerecorded sample of recess play videos, and >80% inter-rater agreement was obtained with an expert assessor (NR) for all SOCARP categories. Social interaction data was not included in the analyses due to the lack of a plausible conceptual association with FMS.

2.3.3. Anthropometrics and Demographics

Body mass (to the nearest 0.1 kg) and stature (to the nearest 0.1 cm) were measured by trained researchers using digital scales and a portable stadiometer, respectively. BMI (kg/m^2) was calculated and converted to zBMI using the 'LMS' method for analysis [51]. Information about children's demographics (i.e., date of birth, gender, ethnicity, home postcode) were provided by parents or guardians within a questionnaire that was returned with the signed consent form. Household postcode was used to classify children into deciles of deprivation level using the English indices of deprivation [48].

2.4. Statistical Analysis

All statistical analysis was undertaken using R open-source software (v.3.6.2., www.r-project.org (accessed on 28 May 2021). A complete case analysis was undertaken (i.e., children with missing demographic, FMS, or SOCARP data were excluded from the analyses). Independent *t*-tests (age, BMI z-score, FMS outcomes), or chi-square tests (deprivation decile, ethnicity) were used to assess differences between those participants who were included and excluded from the final analysis.

A CoDA [46,47,52] was undertaken to examine associations between play behaviors and FMS. In advance, the cmultRepl function within the package zComposition (v.1.3.4) was used to replace zero counts in the play behavior data [53] before an orthogonal isometric logarithmic ratio (Ilr) transformation of the play variables. Descriptive statistics were subsequently calculated for the final sample: this included arithmetic means and standard deviations, geometric means for play behavior composite variables and pairwise variation matrices to show the dispersion of the play behaviors (all calculated using the package 'compositions' v2.0.1). Each SOCARP play behavior category (*activity level*; *activity type*; *group size*) included time-use compositional data which was expressed as Ilr coordinates called pivot coordinates [47,54]. Specifically, *activity level* included five sets of four coordinates (time spent in lying, sitting, standing, walking, and very active); *activity type* included five sets of four coordinates (time spent in active games with equipment, active games without equipment, quiet play, sedentary, and locomotion); and *group size* included four sets of three coordinates (alone, small, medium, and large group).

To examine FMS associations with play behaviors, separate linear regression analyses were undertaken for each play behavior composition, i.e., *activity level*, *activity type*, and *group size*. Models included preschool as a random effect to account for the nesting of participants, and were adjusted for age, sex, and zBMI, but not deprivation, as this did not improve model fit. As a first step, the overall effect of the play behavior category composition was checked using the ANOVA table of model fit. If the play behavior composition was not significantly associated with the FMS outcome, no further analysis was undertaken. If the play behavior composition was significant, separate models were carried out using a different set of pivot coordinates, which encompass the full range of possible combinations of different behaviors relative to all the remaining behaviors in that category. Thus, equivalent statistical models were constructed for each play behavior category (e.g., *activity type*), with each variable within each set sequentially entered as the first Ilr coordinate (i.e., active games with equipment, active games without equipment, sedentary, quiet play, or locomotion), relative to all remaining play behavior variables in that category [46]. Total skill score, object-control, and locomotor skill scores represented the outcome (dependent) variables in the mixed linear regression models (run using the 'stats' package v3.6.2 and lm function), with the first isometric log-ratio coordinates (pivot coordinate) for each play behavior category entered as the explanatory (independent) variable [52]. The isometric log-ratio linear regression models were checked to ensure assumptions were not violated. Significance was set at $p < 0.05$.

3. Results

3.1. Descriptives

Table 1 shows descriptive statistics for the final sample with complete demographic, FMS, and SOCARP data, comprising 133 children aged 3–5 years (55% boys). Compositional variation matrices for play behavior data are in Supplementary file (Tables S1–S3). No significant differences were found for sex, zBMI, deprivation, or ethnicity between those included or excluded from the study, though those included were slightly older ($p < 0.001$). Many of the children (79.7%) lived in areas ranked in the highest decile for deprivation and were predominantly white British (82.7%), with the other children represented as mixed race (4.5%), other white descent (3.8%), Asian (3.8%), Black African (3.8%), or other (1.4%). Almost a quarter of the children (24.8%) were overweight or obese [51].

Table 1. Descriptive statistics for the final sample ($n = 133$).

Variables	Mean (SD)	Geometric Mean
Demographics		
Age (Years)	4.70 (0.53)	-
Body mass index z-scores	0.74 (1.00)	-
Play Behaviors		
Child Activity Level		
Lying (%)	0.73 (3.51)	0.11
Sitting (%)	8.04 (14.50)	3.43
Standing (%)	27.81 (19.01)	28.30
Walking (%)	33.85 (17.02)	40.14
Very Active (%)	29.58 (21.29)	28.02
Activity Type		
Active Games with Equipment (%)	38.24 (38.89)	41.11
Active Games without Equipment (%)	11.44 (20.47)	5.85
Sedentary (%)	14.93 (18.80)	13.60
Quiet Play (%)	8.37 (19.38)	3.23
Locomotion (%)	27.02 (25.08)	36.21
Group Size		
Alone (%)	37.64 (32.86)	33.99
Small (%)	52.49 (31.30)	62.48

Table 1. Cont.

Variables	Mean (SD)	Geometric Mean
Medium (%)	8.97 (19.64)	3.38
Large (%)	0.90 (5.30)	0.15
Foundational Movement Skills		
Total score (range: 0–142 skill components)	63.04 (12.68)	-
Object control skills (range: 0–78 skill components)	29.47 (8.04)	-
Locomotor skills (range: 0–64 skill components)	33.57 (6.74)	-

FMS competence scores were generally low-moderate across the sample, with locomotor scores higher than object-control skill scores. The most frequently observed play behavior activity level among the preschoolers was walking followed by standing and very active behaviors, while children spent less time in sitting and lying. Children therefore spent almost 70% of recess in moderate- to- vigorous-intensity physical activity. Children spent most of recess within small groups or on their own, rather than in medium or large groups. The most common activity types were active play with equipment and locomotion activities, followed by sedentary activities, with limited time spent in active play without equipment and quiet play.

3.2. Compositional Regression Analyses

Table 2 shows a summary of the isometric log-ratio regression models examining play behavior composites and FMS outcomes (total skills, object-control skills, and locomotor skills). Table 3 shows the subsequent further analyses examining the associations between total skill score and locomotor skill score FMS outcomes and play behavior activity type isometric log-ratio regression estimates (pivot coordinates).

Table 2. Isometric log-ratio regression models examining play behavior composites and FMS.

Model	Total Skills Score			Object-Control Skills			Locomotor Skills		
	X^2	df	Pr ($>X^2$)	X^2	df	Pr ($>X^2$)	X^2	df	Pr ($>X^2$)
Activity Level									
Activity Level Ilr	7.66	4	0.105	9.04	4	0.060	3.04	4	0.551
Body mass index	1.51	1	0.219	1.73	1	0.189	0.63	1	0.428
Sex	0.72	1	0.397	10.04	1	0.002 *	4.48	1	0.034 *
Age	19.30	1	0.000 *	16.36	1	0.000 *	12.48	1	0.000 *
Activity Type									
Activity Type Ilr	11.66	4	0.020 *	7.80	4	0.092	9.93	4	0.042 *
Body mass index	3.69	1	0.054	4.00	1	0.046 *	1.47	1	0.225
Sex	0.08	1	0.782	6.85	1	0.009 *	6.27	1	0.012 *
Age	15.32	1	0.000 *	11.55	1	0.001 *	10.06	1	0.002 *
Group Size									
Group Size Ilr	0.84	3	0.840	0.85	3	0.836	1.51	3	0.679
Body mass index	2.81	1	0.093	2.84	1	0.092	1.35	1	0.245
Sex	0.29	1	0.593	7.63	1	0.006 *	5.11	1	0.024 *
Age	15.61	1	0.000 *	13.26	1	0.000 *	10.38	1	0.001 *

Notes. Ilr = play behavior composite variable; X^2 = chi-square value; df = degrees of freedom; Pr ($>X^2$) = probability of observed chi-square statistic that indicates whether the regression coefficient is not equal to zero in the model; * significant association with the FMS outcomes ($p < 0.05$). All models included preschool as a random factor to account for nesting of participants.

Table 3. Summary of associations between FMS outcomes and play behavior activity type isometric log-ratio regression estimates (pivot coordinates).

Model First Pivot Coordinate	Total Skills Score				Locomotor Skills			
	β_1 llr	LCI	UCI	p-Value	β_1 llr	LCI	UCI	p-Value
Activity Type								
(i) Active games with equipment	−0.87	−2.94	1.20	0.412	−0.08	−1.20	1.04	0.884
(ii) Active games without equipment	2.03	0.46	3.60	0.011 *	1.08	0.23	1.93	0.013
(iii) Sedentary	0.51	−1.17	2.20	0.550	0.44	−0.47	1.35	0.342
(iv) Quiet Play	0.13	−1.28	1.55	0.853	0.30	−0.46	1.07	0.438
(v) Locomotion	−2.96	−5.02	−0.89	0.005 *	−1.50	−2.62	−0.37	0.009

Notes. β_1 llr = first isometric log-ratio regression coefficients (pivot coordinate), which should be considered in terms of reallocating time to the behavior relative to the remaining activity type behaviors; LCI: lower 95% confidence interval limit; UCI: upper 95% confidence interval limit. Separate models were run for each set of pivot coordinates. All models included school as a random factor and were adjusted for age, sex, and zBMI.
* Bolded coefficients = significant association with the FMS outcomes ($p < 0.05$).

3.2.1. Total Skills and Play Behaviors

No significant associations were found for *activity level* and *group size* composite estimates with total skills score (Table 2). Therefore, no further analyses were undertaken for these play behavior compositions. *Activity type* was significantly associated with total skills score (Table 2), therefore further analyses were carried out. As shown in Table 3, relative to the other *activity type* behaviors, time spent in active games without equipment was positively associated with the total skills score ($\beta_1 = 2.03$, $p = 0.011$), and time spent in locomotion activities was negatively associated with the total skills score ($\beta_1 = -2.96$, $p = 0.005$).

3.2.2. Object-Control Skills and Play Behaviors

No significant associations were found for *activity level*, *activity type*, and *group size* composite estimates with object-control skills score (Table 2). Therefore, no further analyses were undertaken.

3.2.3. Locomotor Skills and Play Behaviors

No significant associations were found within *activity level* and *group size* composition estimates (Table 2). Therefore, no further analyses were undertaken for these play behavior compositions. *Activity type* was significantly associated with locomotor skills score (Table 2), therefore further analyses were undertaken. As shown in Table 3, relative to the other *activity type* behaviors, active games without equipment were positively associated with locomotor skills ($\beta_1 = 1.08$, $p = 0.013$), and time spent in locomotion was negatively associated with locomotor skills ($\beta_1 = -1.50$, $p = 0.009$).

4. Discussion

This study aimed to examine the relationships between FMS and play behaviors in typically developing preschool children during preschool recess using CoDA. Significant associations were observed within play behavior activity type and FMS. Time spent in active games without equipment, relative to other activity types, was positively associated with higher total skill and locomotor skills scores. Time spent in locomotion (moving while not engaged in an active play game, e.g., transitions from one play activity to the next), relative to the other activity types, was negatively associated with total skill score and locomotor skill score. No associations were observed for activity intensity level or group size play behavior time-use composites with FMS. The findings indicate that participation in specific types of play behaviors during recess are potentially important for FMS development in young children. This is the first study to use CoDA to examine FMS and play behaviors in preschool children, a statistical approach which recognizes that time dependent behaviors (e.g., during recess) are mutually exclusive, as time spent in one behavior can only be changed by concurrently changing one or more other behaviors by the same duration [46,47]. The findings from previous literature are predominantly based on univariate analysis where behaviors are analyzed in isolation from the remaining behaviors [47]. While not directly comparable to the present study, these studies are incorporated into the discussion to facilitate the interpretation and explanation of the results.

A key finding in the present study was that time spent in active games without equipment, relative to the other activity types, was positively associated with total and locomotor FMS scores. Though, on average, children in our sample spent limited time in this type of activity, this finding suggests that spending more time on active games without equipment such as dancing, hide and seek, chasing games, imaginative play, rough and tumble, as well as verbal games that involve actions and clapping (e.g., ring-a-roses), may be important for FMS development. Alternatively, children with high FMS competence spend a higher proportion of their recess playtime participating in active games without equipment. It can be expected that these activities are related to locomotor skills, as running, hopping, jumping, leaping, galloping, and sliding are frequently utilized in these types of play. Previous research has demonstrated that participation in dance activities during the preschool day is positively associated with locomotor skill development in young children [55]. However, counterintuitively, no relationship was observed in the study between frequency of walking or running activities and locomotor skills [55]. The present study included locomotion as an activity type, which represented children engaged in a locomotor activity (e.g., walking, jogging, running, skipping without a rope) that *was not* part of a sport or active game, such as while transitioning from one activity to the next. These locomotion activities were negatively associated with total and locomotor skill scores. This may represent children that are on the periphery of participating in active game play and struggling to find an engaging and meaningful play activity that might support skill development—a phenomena described by Herrington and Brussoni as 'channel surfing' [56]. These children may require encouragement and need to be offered a range of possibilities to substitute this locomotion activity with more active forms of play. Indeed, it is possible that simply moving or transitioning from one place to another without an active play purpose may not be sufficient to foster FMS; meaningful, playful locomotor activities may be necessary needed to acquire skills.

On average, children spent a relatively large proportion of recess time (41%) engaged in active games with equipment, yet greater time spent in this type of play behavior was not associated with FMS. This may suggest that the fixed and portable (loose parts) equipment available in these preschool settings did not provide children with the affordances for locomotor and object-control skill development. Like Tsuda et al., who examined FMS and physical activity during free play in two preschools [57], our observations revealed that limited bats and balls were available during recess for children to practice object-control skills. Children were frequently observed idly sitting on wheeled toys or aboard fixed climbing structures. It is possible that these pieces of equipment supported other FMS capacities, such as lower body strength, climbing, or stability skills, not assessed in the present study. Nevertheless, our finding is similar to previous research that reported that different types of playground design and equipment involved a limited number of FMS [58]. A systematic review examining the value of playgrounds for children's physical activity levels found that the presence of a fixed structure athletics track was positively associated with physical activity, while the availability of slides, sandboxes, and swinging equipment on the playground—all of which can involve turn-taking—were negatively associated with activity levels [59]. Other studies have found less fixed or static playground equipment and more portable play equipment (e.g., balls, portable slides) to be beneficial for young children's physical activity levels [60–62]. While this suggests that upgrading the type and volume of portable equipment in preschools could assist with engaging children in playful activities that facilitate the development of object-control skills (e.g., providing a wide variety and number of balls in different sizes and colors), it is recommended that future research examines the association between FMS and fixed versus portable equipment separately. It is important to note that the above-mentioned studies investigated physical activity levels rather than FMS and focused on the presence of equipment in the playground, rather than children's engagement in active games using the equipment like in the current study. Nevertheless, these studies and others highlight numerous preschool and playground environmental characteristics that contribute to children's activity levels at preschool such as larger playground size, presence of an open field with no markings, and fewer children on the playground [59]. Thus, given that physical activity drives FMS development in the early years [2], further research examining the influence of preschool physical environmental characteristics and the volume and type of fixed and portable equipment on active play and FMS is warranted.

Geometric means indicated that participants in this study spent relatively greater recess time in moderate- to- vigorous physical activity, comprising walking (40%) and very active behaviors (28%). Recess periods in preschool are shorter and more frequent, and there is evidence that this leads to increased moderate- to- vigorous physical activity [39,63], which may explain the very active physical activity levels observed. However, findings showed that the activity intensity play behavior composite mean was not associated with preschoolers' FMS. This finding is somewhat inconsistent with recent evidence from two systematic reviews that found positive associations between physical activity levels and FMS among young children, including at moderate- and- vigorous intensities [23,24]—inclusive of the results from our own research [22], which involved the same sample of children involved in the current study. Our study and others included in the systematic reviews examined habitual physical activity and FMS. Results from studies examining FMS and young children's physical activity during preschool hours and specifically preschool recess are mixed. For example, Iivonen et al. [64] directly observed physical activity during three consecutive preschool days in a small sample of Finnish children (n = 53) and found that light and moderate-to-vigorous physical activity were not associated with FMS. In contrast, Tsuda et al. [57] examined physical activity using accelerometers during free-play time at preschool (i.e., recess) in a cross-sectional study and reported that locomotor and object-control skills significantly predicted moderate- to- vigorous physical activity (n.b., the authors did not examine FMS as the dependent variable). To cloud the issue further, there is evidence that suggests that low intensity activities at preschool are associated with FMS. Martins et al. recently demonstrated through accelerometry and CoDA that increasing sedentary time at the expense of light physical activity elicited improved manipulative skills in preschool children [65]. In relation, Butcher and Eaton [66] found that 5-year-old children who participated in low intensity, fine motor activities during indoor free play were more likely to have good visual motor control and balance. Taken together, these diverse results indicate that more research is needed to examine the relationship between activity intensity and FMS during preschool, and specifically during recess. Studies that capture information about the types and context of physical activity during recess alongside the intensity of movement are needed to better understand the nature of playful skill development.

No associations were observed for group size play behavior composites with FMS. On average, children spent a relatively large proportion of recess time playing alone or in small groups. Neither individual or group activity was found to be important for FMS, but this may change over time as children's social and emotional skills develop and their play preferences mature from solitary play to complex social play [19,67]. For example, ball skills may be augmented through small-sided games as children progress to more stereotypical playground activities in primary school that involve larger group sizes such as football. We did not examine whether the composition of groups (e.g., same sex versus mixed), teacher involvement, or teacher proximity to child play activities were associated with preschoolers' FMS development. Herrmann et al. [19] have described how young children tend to make friends with the same gender. Furthermore, boys engage in more individual play and girls more frequently engage in cooperative play. Thus, gender differences in play group compositions may influence FMS. Previous studies have also shown how childcare educators' education, attitudes, beliefs, behaviors, and practices may influence preschool children's physical activity, FMS, and physical literacy [68–70]. Therefore, examining if and how teacher attitudes and practices in relation to play behaviors and FMS and how teacher interactions with children during recess affect FMS competence could be an interesting area for future study.

The purpose of the current study was to better understand how young children's preschool recess play behaviors are related to FMS competence. Under the United Nations Convention on the Rights of the Child, children have the right to play [71]. It is important to emphasize that the authors' position is that recess play should remain play, i.e., freely chosen, purposeless, self-directed, and intrinsically motivated [29–31]. Though we were interested in play and FMS development, we consider that play is an end in itself [56], and recess play to be a context for activities that are unstructured and fun. We also recognize that play is a diverse and complex behavior that is essential for child development [72]. Thus, we are not advocating for adult-directed, structured FMS programs during preschool recess, for example, to deliver active games without equipment. Rather, preschool settings and educators should seek to maximize the opportunities for young children to engage in diverse active play experiences [73]. The environmental resources available to each child to foster FMS could be enhanced through changing the design of play spaces within the recess playground to include natural landscapes and features (e.g., forested areas with trees and shrubs, rocks, water, sand, uneven ground, slopes) [56,74,75], as well as increasing the volume and range of loose parts and fixed equipment [60–62]. The role of preschool educators should be to encourage and offer possibilities for active play while fully respecting child agency [68–70]. Nevertheless, due to the narrow evidence base, more research exploring how to maximize affordances for young children to develop FMS during preschool recess periods is warranted.

The strengths of this study include the use of direct observation and video assessments of FMS and play behaviors, which ensured that information about the quality of FMS movements and types of play behaviors (rather than just activity levels) were captured. Furthermore, recruitment included a representative sample from northwest England, which is more deprived than other parts of the country. A major strength is the use of compositional data analyses to consider the time dependent nature of the play behavior data to examine the associations between play behaviors, relative to one another, with FMS. The limitations of the study include a lack of generalizability of the study findings due to the primarily disadvantaged and regional sample. Further, play behavior data was captured through 5-min observations. Longer observation periods may have captured more diverse play behaviors. In addition, the time of day of the recess periods might have also influenced play behaviors but was not computed for use in the analysis. Furthermore, there was a high proportion of missing data as feasibility constraints meant that SOCARP measurements could only be captured in a sub-sample of children, while the total number FMS assessments were limited by absent children or missing skills due to technical issues. Furthermore, capturing information about the environmental characteristics and policies in preschool settings that may influence FMS affordances and physical activity (such as through the Environmental and Policy Assessment and Observation Tool: EPAO [76]) would have facilitated a deeper understanding and stronger interpretation of the study findings had they been measured and controlled for. Similarly, SOCARP captures broad activity types and coding play behaviors in a more detailed way, such as using the recently developed Tool for Observing Play Outdoors (TOPO) [77], may help to facilitate a more detailed understanding of the association between play activity types and FMS, such as the specific and different types of active games with and without equipment. Finally, the study only included assessments of locomotor and object-control FMS. Had a broader range of FMS assessments been used, such as stability and fine motor skills as well as broader FMS such as strength or cycling, more associations with play behaviors could have been uncovered.

5. Conclusions

In conclusion, significant associations were found within the play behavior activity type compositions: relatively more time spent in active games without equipment were associated with higher total and locomotor FMS scores, while relatively more time in locomotion activities was associated with lower total and locomotor FMS scores. No associations were found between activity level and group size play behavior compositions and FMS. The findings indicate that participation in specific play behaviors during recess may be important for FMS development in young children, though we are unable to draw causal conclusions. Future research, including longitudinal data, is required to confirm and expand these findings.

Supplementary Materials: The following are available online at https://www.mdpi.com/article/10.3390/children8070543/s1, Table S1: Table reporting variation matrices of time spent in different activity levels; Table S2: Table reporting variation matrices of time spent in different group sizes; Table S3: Table reporting variation matrices of time spent in different activity types.

Author Contributions: Conceptualization, L.F.; methodology, G.S., L.F., M.V.O. and N.D.R.; formal analysis, M.V.O., J.D.F. and M.C.; validation; L.F., N.D.R. and T.U.; investigation, L.F., M.V.O. and N.D.R.; data curation, M.C.; writing—original draft preparation, L.F. and M.C.; writing—review and editing, M.C., J.D.F., S.J.F., Z.R.K., N.D.R., G.S. and T.U.; supervision, G.S. and L.F.; project administration G.S. and L.F.; funding acquisition, G.S. All authors have read and agreed to the published version of the manuscript.

Funding: This research was funded by the Neighbourhood Renewal Fund and Liverpool John Moores University.

Institutional Review Board Statement: The study was conducted in accordance with the guidelines of the Declaration of Helsinki and was approved by the University Research Ethics Committee of Liverpool John Moores University (protocol code 09/SPS/027; date of approval: 2 September 2009).

Informed Consent Statement: Informed consent from parents/guardians and child assent was obtained from all participants involved in the study.

Data Availability Statement: The data presented in this study are available upon request from the corresponding author. The data are not publicly available due to ethical approval restrictions.

Acknowledgments: Liz Lamb at Sportslinx/Liverpool City Council, the active play management (Pam Stevenson) and delivery team (Richard Jones, Adam Tinsley, and Julie Walker), the Liverpool Early Years Team and the LJMU Physical Activity, Exercise and Health research group work bank volunteers who assisted with data collection. We would also like to thank the schools, children's centres, and families who participated in the study.

Conflicts of Interest: The authors declare no conflict of interest. The funders had no role in the design of the study; in the collection, analyses, or interpretation of data; in the writing of the manuscript; or in the decision to publish the results.

References

1. Hulteen, R.M.; Morgan, P.J.; Barnett, L.M.; Stodden, D.F.; Lubans, D.R. Development of Foundational Movement Skills: A Conceptual Model for Physical Activity Across the Lifespan. *Sports Med.* **2018**, *48*, 1533–1540. [CrossRef]
2. Stodden, D.F.; Goodway, J.D.; Langendorfer, S.J.; Roberton, M.A.; Rudisill, M.E.; Garcia, C.; Garcia, L.E. A Developmental Perspective on the Role of Motor Skill Competence in Physical Activity: An Emergent Relationship. *Quest* **2008**, *60*, 290–306. [CrossRef]
3. Gallahue, D.L.; Ozmun, J.C.; Goodway, J. *Understanding Motor Development: Infants, Children, Adolescents, Adults*, 7th ed.; McGraw-Hill Education: New York, NY, USA, 2012.
4. Foulkes, J.D.; Knowles, Z.; Fairclough, S.J.; Stratton, G.; O'Dwyer, M.; Ridgers, N.D.; Foweather, L. Fundamental Movement skills of preschool children in Northwest England. *Percept. Mot. Ski.* **2015**, *121*, 260–283. [CrossRef] [PubMed]
5. Dobell, A.; Pringle, A.; Faghy, M.A.; Roscoe, C.M.P. Fundamental Movement Skills and Accelerometer-Measured Physical Activity Levels during Early Childhood: A Systematic Review. *Children* **2020**, *7*, 224. [CrossRef]
6. Newell, K. Constraints in the development of coordination. In *Motor Developmnet in Children: Aspects of Coordination and Control*; Wade, M., Whiting, H., Eds.; Martinus Nijhoff Publishers: Dordrecht, The Netherlands, 1986; pp. 341–360.
7. Clark, J.E.; Metcalfe, J.S. The Mountain of Motor Development: A Metaphor. In *Motor Development: Research and Reviews*; Clark, J.E., Humphrey, J., Eds.; NASPE Publications: Reston, VA, USA, 2002; Volume 2, pp. 163–190.
8. Tyler, R.; Mackintosh, K.A.; Foweather, L.; Edwards, L.C.; Stratton, G. Youth motor competence promotion model: A quantitative investigation into modifiable factors. *J. Sci. Med. Sport* **2020**, *23*, 955–961. [CrossRef]

9. Gallahue, D.L.; Cleland-donnelly, F. *Developmental Physical Education for all Children + Journal Access*; Human Kinetics: Champaign, IL, USA, 2003.
10. Lima, R.A.; Pfeiffer, K.; Larsen, L.R.; Bugge, A.; Moller, N.C.; Anderson, L.B.; Stodden, D.F. Physical Activity and Motor Competence Present a Positive Reciprocal Longitudinal Relationship Across Childhood and Early Adolescence. *J. Phys. Act. Health* **2017**, *14*, 440–447. [CrossRef]
11. De Meester, A.; Stodden, D.; Goodway, J.; True, L.; Brian, A.; Ferkel, R.; Haerens, L. Identifying a motor proficiency barrier for meeting physical activity guidelines in children. *J. Sci. Med. Sport* **2018**, *21*, 58–62. [CrossRef] [PubMed]
12. Seefeldt, V. Developmental motor patterns: Implications for elementary school physical education. In *Psychology of Motor Behavior and Sport*; Nadeau, C.H., Halliwell, W.R., Newell, K., Roberts, G., Eds.; Human Kinetics: Champaign, IL, USA, 1979; pp. 314–323.
13. Loprinzi, P.D.; Davis, R.E.; Fu, Y.-C. Early motor skill competence as a mediator of child and adult physical activity. *Prev. Med. Rep.* **2015**, *2*, 833–838. [CrossRef]
14. Vlahov, E.; Baghurst, T.M.; Mwavita, M. Preschool motor development predicting high school health-related physical fitness: A prospective study. *Percept. Mot. Ski.* **2014**, *119*, 279–291. [CrossRef]
15. Pagani, L.S.; Messier, S. Links between Motor Skills and Indicators of School Readiness at Kindergarten Entry in Urban Disadvantaged Children. *J. Educ. Dev. Psychol.* **2012**, *2*, 95. [CrossRef]
16. Piek, J.P.; Dawson, L.; Smith, L.M.; Gasson, N. The role of early fine and gross motor development on later motor and cognitive ability. *Hum. Mov. Sci.* **2008**, *27*, 668–681. [CrossRef] [PubMed]
17. van der Fels, I.M.; Te Wierike, S.C.; Hartman, E.; Elferink-Gemser, M.T.; Smith, J.; Visscher, C. The relationship between motor skills and cognitive skills in 4–16 year old typically developing children: A systematic review. *J. Sci. Med. Sport* **2015**, *18*, 697–703. [CrossRef] [PubMed]
18. Gonzalez, S.L.; Alvarez, V.; Nelson, E.L. Do Gross and Fine Motor Skills Differentially Contribute to Language Outcomes? A Systematic Review. *Front. Psychol.* **2019**, *10*, 2670. [CrossRef] [PubMed]
19. Herrmann, C.; Bretz, K.; Kuhnis, J.; Seelig, H.; Keller, R.; Ferrari, I. Connection between Social Relationships and Basic Motor Competencies in Early Childhood. *Children* **2021**, *8*, 53. [CrossRef]
20. Logan, S.W.; Scrabis-Fletcher, K.; Modlesky, C.; Getchell, N. The relationship between motor skill proficiency and body mass index in preschool children. *Res. Q. Exerc. Sport* **2011**, *82*, 442–448. [CrossRef]
21. Duncan, M.J.; Hall, C.; Eyre, E.; Barnett, L.M.; James, R.S. Pre-schoolers fundamental movement skills predict BMI, physical activity, and sedentary behavior: A longitudinal study. *Scand. J. Med. Sci. Sports* **2021**, *31* (Suppl. 1), 8–14. [CrossRef]
22. Foweather, L.; Knowles, Z.; Ridgers, N.D.; O'Dwyer, M.V.; Foulkes, J.D.; Stratton, G. Fundamental movement skills in relation to weekday and weekend physical activity in preschool children. *J. Sci. Med. Sport* **2015**, *18*, 691–696. [CrossRef]
23. Jones, D.; Innerd, A.; Giles, E.L.; Azevedo, L.B. Association between fundamental motor skills and physical activity in the early years: A systematic review and meta-analysis. *J. Sport Health Sci.* **2020**, *9*, 542–552. [CrossRef]
24. Xin, F.; Chen, S.T.; Clark, C.; Hong, J.T.; Liu, Y.; Cai, Y.J. Relationship between Fundamental Movement Skills and Physical Activity in Preschool-Aged Children: A Systematic Review. *Int. J. Environ. Res. Public Health* **2020**, *17*, 3566. [CrossRef]
25. Trevlas, E.; Matsouka, O.; Zachopoulou, E. Relationship between playfulness and motor creativity in preschool children. *Early Child. Dev. Care* **2003**, *173*, 535–543. [CrossRef]
26. Pellegrini, A.D.; Smith, P.K. Physical activity play: The nature and function of a neglected aspect of playing. *Child. Dev.* **1998**, *69*, 577–598. [CrossRef] [PubMed]
27. Pellegrini, A.D.; Smith, P.K. The Development of Play During Childhood: Forms and Possible Functions. *Child. Adolesc. Ment. Health* **1998**, *3*, 51–57. [CrossRef]
28. Pellegrini, A.D.; Dupuis, D.; Smith, P.K. Play in evolution and development. *Dev. Rev.* **2007**, *27*, 261–276. [CrossRef]
29. Morrison, C.D.; Bundy, A.C.; Fisher, A.G. The contribution of motor skills and playfulness to the play performance of preschoolers. *Am. J. Occup. Ther.* **1991**, *45*, 687–694. [CrossRef]
30. O'Grady, M.G.; Dusing, S.C. Reliability and validity of play-based assessments of motor and cognitive skills for infants and young children: A systematic review. *Phys. Ther.* **2015**, *95*, 25–38. [CrossRef] [PubMed]
31. Perimutter, J.C.; Pellegrini, A.D. Children's verbal fantasy play with parents and peers. *Educ. Psych.* **1987**, *7*, 269–281. [CrossRef]
32. Bjorklund, D.F.; Brown, R.D. Physical play and cognitive development: Integrating activity, cognition, and education. *Child. Dev.* **1998**, *69*, 604–606. [CrossRef]
33. Burdette, H.L.; Whitaker, R.C. Resurrecting free play in young children: Looking beyond fitness and fatness to attention, affiliation, and affect. *Arch. Pediatr. Adolesc. Med.* **2005**, *159*, 46–50. [CrossRef] [PubMed]
34. Veiga, G.; Leng, W.D.; Cachucho, R.; Ketelaar, L.; Kok, J.N.; Knobbe, A.; Neto, C.; Rieffe, C. Social Competence at the Playground: Preschoolers During Recess. *Inf. Child. Dev.* **2017**, *26*, e1957. [CrossRef]
35. Timmons, B.W.; Leblanc, A.G.; Carson, V.; Connor Gorber, S.; Dillman, C.; Janssen, I.; Kho, M.E.; Spence, J.C.; Stearns, J.A.; Tremblay, M.S. Systematic review of physical activity and health in the early years (aged 0–4 years). *Appl. Physiol. Nutr. Metab.* **2012**, *37*, 773–792. [CrossRef]
36. Truelove, S.; Vanderloo, L.M.; Tucker, P. Defining and Measuring Active Play among Young Children: A Systematic Review. *J. Phys. Act. Health* **2017**, *14*, 155–166. [CrossRef] [PubMed]
37. Tovey, H. Playing on the edge: Perceptions of risk and danger in outdoor play. In *Play and Learning in the Early Years*; Broadhead, P., Howard, J., Wood, E., Eds.; SAGE: London, UK, 2010; pp. 79–94.

38. Bento, G.; Dias, G. The importance of outdoor play for young children's healthy development. *Porto Biomed. J.* **2017**, *2*, 157–160. [CrossRef] [PubMed]
39. Tandon, P.S.; Saelens, B.E.; Zhou, C.; Christakis, D.A. A Comparison of Preschoolers' Physical Activity Indoors versus Outdoors at Child Care. *Int. J. Environ. Res. Public Health* **2018**, *15*, 2463. [CrossRef]
40. Iivonen, S.; Sääkslahti, A.K. Preschool children's fundamental motor skills: A review of significant determinants. *Early Child. Dev. Care* **2014**, *184*, 1107–1126. [CrossRef]
41. Barnett, L.M.; Lai, S.K.; Veldman, S.L.C.; Hardy, L.L.; Cliff, D.P.; Morgan, P.J.; Zask, A.; Lubans, D.R.; Shultz, S.P.; Ridgers, N.D.; et al. Correlates of Gross Motor Competence in Children and Adolescents: A Systematic Review and Meta-Analysis. *Sports Med.* **2016**, *46*, 1663–1688. [CrossRef]
42. Organisation for Economic Co-operation and Development PF3.2: Enrolment in Childcare and Pre-School. Available online: https://www.oecd.org/els/soc/PF3_2_Enrolment_childcare_preschool.pdf (accessed on 29 May 2021).
43. Department for Education Statutory Framework for the Early Years Foundation Stage. Available online: https://assets.publishing.service.gov.uk/government/uploads/system/uploads/attachment_data/file/596629/EYFS_STATUTORY_FRAMEWORK_2017.pdf (accessed on 29 May 2021).
44. O'Dwyer, M.; Fairclough, S.J.; Ridgers, N.D.; Knowles, Z.R.; Foweather, L.; Stratton, G. Patterns of objectively measured moderate-to-vigorous physical activity in preschool children. *J. Phys. Act. Health* **2014**, *11*, 1233–1238. [CrossRef] [PubMed]
45. True, L.; Pfeiffer, K.A.; Dowda, M.; Williams, H.G.; Brown, W.H.; O'Neill, J.R.; Pate, R.R. Motor competence and characteristics within the preschool environment. *J. Sci. Med. Sport* **2017**, *20*, 751–755. [CrossRef]
46. Chastin, S.F.; Palarea-Albaladejo, J.; Dontje, M.L.; Skelton, D.A. Combined Effects of Time Spent in Physical Activity, Sedentary Behaviors and Sleep on Obesity and Cardio-Metabolic Health Markers: A Novel Compositional Data Analysis Approach. *PLoS ONE* **2015**, *10*, e0139984. [CrossRef]
47. Dumuid, D.; Pedisic, Z.; Palarea-Albaladejo, J.; Martin-Fernandez, J.A.; Hron, K.; Olds, T. Compositional Data Analysis in Time-Use Epidemiology: What, Why, How. *Int. J. Environ. Res. Public Health* **2020**, *17*, 2220. [CrossRef]
48. Department for Communities and Local Government, UK Government. The English Indices of Deprivation 2010. Available online: https://www.gov.uk/government/statistics/english-indices-of-deprivation-2010 (accessed on 21 June 2021).
49. Williams, H.G.; Pfeiffer, K.A.; Dowda, M.; Jeter, C.; Jones, S.; Pate, R.R. A Field-Based Testing Protocol for Assessing Gross Motor Skills in Preschool Children: The CHAMPS Motor Skills Protocol (CMSP). *Meas. Phys. Educ. Exerc. Sci.* **2009**, *13*, 151–165. [CrossRef]
50. Ridgers, N.D.; Stratton, G.; McKenzie, T.L. Reliability and validity of the System for Observing Children's Activity and Relationships during Play (SOCARP). *J. Phys. Act. Health* **2010**, *7*, 17–25. [CrossRef]
51. Cole, T.J.; Lobstein, T. Extended international (IOTF) body mass index cut-offs for thinness, overweight and obesity. *Pediatr. Obes.* **2012**, *7*, 284–294. [CrossRef]
52. Hron, K.; Filzmoser, P.; Thompson, K. Linear regression with compositional explanatory variables. *J. Appl. Stat.* **2012**, *39*, 1115–1128. [CrossRef]
53. Martín-Fernández, J.-A.; Hron, K.; Templ, M.; Filzmoser, P.; Palarea-Albaladejo, J. Bayesian-multiplicative treatment of count zeros in compositional data sets. *Stat. Model.* **2014**, *15*, 134–158. [CrossRef]
54. Muller, I.; Hron, K.; Fiserova, E.; Smahaj, J.; Cakirpaloglu, P.; Vancakova, J. Interpretation of Compositional Regression with Application to Time Budget Analysis. *Austrian J. Stat.* **2018**, *47*, 3–19. [CrossRef]
55. O'Neill, J.R.; Williams, H.G.; Pfeiffer, K.A.; Dowda, M.; McIver, K.L.; Brown, W.H.; Pate, R.R. Young children's motor skill performance: Relationships with activity types and parent perception of athletic competence. *J. Sci. Med. Sport* **2014**, *17*, 607–610. [CrossRef] [PubMed]
56. Herrington, S.; Brussoni, M. Beyond Physical Activity: The Importance of Play and Nature-Based Play Spaces for Children's Health and Development. *Curr. Obes. Rep.* **2015**, *4*, 477–483. [CrossRef]
57. Tsuda, E.; Goodway, J.D.; Famelia, R.; Brian, A. Relationship Between Fundamental Motor Skill Competence, Perceived Physical Competence and Free-Play Physical Activity in Children. *Res. Q. Exerc. Sport* **2020**, *91*, 55–63. [CrossRef]
58. Adams, J.; Barnett, L.; Veitch, J. What sort of playground design facilitates physical activity and encourages children to use diverse motor skills? *J. Sci. Med. Sport* **2018**, *21*, S12. [CrossRef]
59. Broekhuizen, K.; Scholten, A.M.; de Vries, S.I. The value of (pre)school playgrounds for children's physical activity level: A systematic review. *Int. J. Behav. Nutr. Phys. Act.* **2014**, *11*, 59. [CrossRef]
60. Ng, M.; Rosenberg, M.; Thornton, A.; Lester, L.; Trost, S.G.; Bai, P.; Christian, H. The Effect of Upgrades to Childcare Outdoor Spaces on Preschoolers' Physical Activity: Findings from a Natural Experiment. *Int. J. Environ. Res. Public Health* **2020**, *17*, 468. [CrossRef]
61. Dowda, M.; Brown, W.H.; McIver, K.L.; Pfeiffer, K.A.; O'Neill, J.R.; Addy, C.L.; Pate, R.R. Policies and characteristics of the preschool environment and physical activity of young children. *Pediatrics* **2009**, *123*, e261–e266. [CrossRef]
62. Brown, W.H.; Pfeiffer, K.A.; McIver, K.L.; Dowda, M.; Addy, C.L.; Pate, R.R. Social and environmental factors associated with preschoolers' nonsedentary physical activity. *Child. Dev.* **2009**, *80*, 45–58. [CrossRef]
63. Razak, L.A.; Yoong, S.L.; Wiggers, J.; Morgan, P.J.; Jones, J.; Finch, M.; Sutherland, R.; Lecathelnais, C.; Gillham, K.; Clinton-McHarg, T.; et al. Impact of scheduling multiple outdoor free-play periods in childcare on child moderate-to-vigorous physical activity: A cluster randomised trial. *Int. J. Behav. Nutr. Phys. Act.* **2018**, *15*, 34. [CrossRef]

64. Iivonen, S.; Sääkslahti, A.K.; Mehtälä, A.; Villberg, J.J.; Soini, A.; Poskiparta, M. Directly observed physical activity and fundamental motor skills in four-year-old children in day care. *Eur. Early Child. Educ. Res. J.* **2016**, *24*, 398–413. [CrossRef]
65. Martins, C.M.L.; Clark, C.C.T.; Tassitano, R.M.; Filho, A.N.S.; Gaya, A.R.; Duncan, M.J. School-Time Movement Behaviors and Fundamental Movement Skills in Preschoolers: An Isotemporal Reallocation Analysis. *Percept. Mot. Ski.* **2021**. [CrossRef] [PubMed]
66. Butcher, J.E.; Eaton, W.O. Gross and fine motor proficiency in preschoolers: Relationships with free play behaviour and activity level. *J. Hum. Mov. Stud.* **1989**, *16*, 27–36.
67. de Valk, L.; Bekker, T.; Eggen, B. Designing for Social Interaction in Open-Ended Play Environments. *Int. J. Des.* **2015**, *9*, 1.
68. Tonge, K.L.; Jones, R.A.; Okely, A.D. Quality Interactions in Early Childhood Education and Care Center Outdoor Environments. *Early Child. Educ. J.* **2018**, *47*, 31–41. [CrossRef]
69. Foulkes, J.D.; Foweather, L.; Fairclough, S.J.; Knowles, Z. "I Wasn't Sure What It Meant to be Honest"-Formative Research towards a Physical Literacy Intervention for Preschoolers. *Children* **2020**, *7*, 76. [CrossRef]
70. Roscoe, C.M.P.; James, R.S.; Duncan, M.J. Preschool staff and parents' perceptions of preschool children's physical activity and fundamental movement skills from an area of high deprivation: A qualitative study. *Qual. Res. Sport Exerc. Health* **2017**, *9*, 619–635. [CrossRef]
71. United Nations Human Rights Office of the Commissioner: Convention on the Rights of the Child. 1989. Available online: https://www.ohchr.org/EN/ProfessionalInterest/Pages/CRC.aspx (accessed on 20 June 2021).
72. Yogman, M.; Garner, A.; Hutchinson, J.; Hirsh-Pasek, K.; Golinkoff, R.M.; Committee on Psychosocial Aspects of Child and Family Health and Council on Communications and Media. The Power of Play: A Pediatric Role in Enhancing Development in Young Children. *Pediatrics* **2018**, *142*, e20182058. [CrossRef] [PubMed]
73. Heft, H. Affordances of children's environments: A functional approach to environmental description. *Child. Environ. Q.* **1988**, *5*, 29–37.
74. Fjørtoft, I. The Natural Environment as a Playground for Children: The Impact of Outdoor Play Activities in Pre-Primary School Children. *Early Child. Educ. J.* **2001**, *29*, 111–117. [CrossRef]
75. Bjørgen, K. Physical activity in light of affordances in outdoor environments: Qualitative observation studies of 3–5 years olds in kindergarten. *SpringerPlus* **2016**, *5*, 950. [CrossRef] [PubMed]
76. Ward, D.S.; Mazzucca, S.; McWilliams, C.; Hales, D. Use of the Environment and Policy Evaluation and Observation as a Self-Report Instrument (EPAO-SR) to measure nutrition and physical activity environments in child care settings: Validity and reliability evidence. *Int. J. Behav. Nutr. Phys. Act.* **2015**, *12*, 124. [CrossRef]
77. Loebach, J.; Cox, A. Tool for Observing Play Outdoors (TOPO): A New Typology for Capturing Children's Play Behaviors in Outdoor Environments. *Int. J. Environ. Res. Public Health* **2020**, *17*, 5611. [CrossRef]

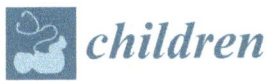

Article

The Effect of Short-Term Wingate-Based High Intensity Interval Training on Anaerobic Power and Isokinetic Muscle Function in Adolescent Badminton Players

Duk-Han Ko [1], Yong-Chul Choi [2] and Dong-Soo Lee [3],*

[1] Department of Sports Science Convergence, Dongguk University, Seoul 04620, Korea; kodh119@hanmail.net
[2] Department of Physical Education, Gangneung-Wonju National University, Gangneung 25457, Korea; skicyc@gwnu.ac.kr
[3] Lee Dong Soo Badminton Academy, Seoul 06548, Korea
* Correspondence: dongsoo74@hanmail.net; Tel.: +82-33-640-2556; Fax: +82-33-641-2878

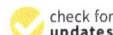

Citation: Ko, D.-H.; Choi, Y.-C.; Lee, D.-S. The Effect of Short-Term Wingate-Based High Intensity Interval Training on Anaerobic Power and Isokinetic Muscle Function in Adolescent Badminton Players. Children 2021, 8, 458. https://doi.org/10.3390/children8060458

Academic Editor: Zoe Knowles

Received: 28 April 2021
Accepted: 26 May 2021
Published: 31 May 2021

Publisher's Note: MDPI stays neutral with regard to jurisdictional claims in published maps and institutional affiliations.

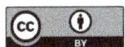

Copyright: © 2021 by the authors. Licensee MDPI, Basel, Switzerland. This article is an open access article distributed under the terms and conditions of the Creative Commons Attribution (CC BY) license (https://creativecommons.org/licenses/by/4.0/).

Abstract: Badminton requires both aerobic fitness and anaerobic ability for high performance. High intensity interval training (HIIT) is a traditional training method for improving fitness. In this study, we investigated whether short-term Wingate-based HIIT is effective for improving anaerobic activity in youth badminton players. Participants included 32 total badminton players in middle school and high school. They were divided into two groups (HIIT and moderate continuous training (MCT)). Training occurred for 4 weeks in total, three times a week, for 30 min each session. A body composition test, isokinetic knee muscle function test (60°/s, 240°/s), Wingate anaerobic power test (30 s × 5 sets), and analysis of heart rate changes were undertaken before and after training. After 4 weeks, body fat decreased in the HIIT group ($p = 0.019$); they also showed superior anaerobic ability compared to the MCT group. Differences were statistically significant in 3–4 sets (three sets, $p = 0.019$; four sets, $p = 0.021$). Regarding fatigue, the HIIT group showed superior fatigue improvement after training and better fatigue recovery ability in 3~5 sets (three sets, $p = 0.032$; four sets, $p = 0.017$; five sets, $p = 0.003$) than the MCT group. Neither group exhibited changes in heart rate during the anaerobic power test after training. Both groups improved in terms of isokinetic knee muscle function at 60°/s with no differences. However, at 240°/s, the HIIT group showed a statistically significant improvement ($p = 0.035$). Therefore, HIIT for 4 weeks improved the athletes' performance and physical strength.

Keywords: badminton; short-term training; high-intensity interval training; adolescent anaerobic

1. Introduction

Badminton is a very popular sport globally. According to the International Olympic Committee (IOC) and the World Badminton Federation, more than 200 million people in the world enjoy this sport. Badminton requires the high-intensity use of the joints for various actions that take place in a short time in a rectangular court [1]. It also requires a high level of physical fitness, as athletes are given only short breaks between matches [2]. The physical factors that affect badminton performance include not only cardiorespiratory endurance, agility, and quickness, but also anaerobic power [3]. In particular, repetitive jumps, continuous rallying, and the agility necessary for changes in movement direction are required in order to traverse large areas of the court very quickly [4]. Therefore, for badminton players, VO2 max is an important factor in determining athletes' performance [5]. In addition, anaerobic ability is required in badminton to perform the necessary intermittent, rapid, and accurate movements while maintaining balance [6]. Sports drills that require frequent long steps after repeated smashing or stopping may offer better performance for athletes with higher functional capacity [7]. In badminton games, about 60–70% of the game uses an aerobic energy substrate, leaving about 30–40% using an anaerobic energy substrate [4]. The aerobic energy substrate refers to the process of synthesizing ATP by introducing the ingested nutrients into the mitochondria, and the anaerobic energy substrate refers to a state that does not require oxygen to generate energy. Previously, various training methods have been applied to improve anaerobic power. One of these methods is high-intensity interval training (HIIT). HIIT is an interval-based form of exercise that maintains more than 80% of the maximum oxygen intake. In many reports, HIIT has been found to be the best way to improve aerobic and anaerobic capacity. Its benefits also appear more quickly than those of traditional training methods [8,9]. Therefore, HIIT has been commonly used for the training of athletes since the 1950s [10]. It is designed to increase the lactate and anaerobic thresholds through repeating periods of high intensity and rest [11]. HIIT has been used by many athletes to develop their ability to recover quickly during short breaks [12]. Training has been reported to be effective when it is conducted for 8–12 weeks, and some studies have indicated that there was a significant improvement with 2–6-week periods of HIIT [13,14]. Despite its positive effects, HIIT has a high risk of adverse effects and dropout in children and adolescents with low fitness levels because it repeats and sustains high-intensity bouts of 80% or more of the maximum oxygen intake [15]. As a result of meta-analysis on dropout of HIIT in previous studies, consisting of an analysis of 1318 people in total, HIIT dropout accounted for 17.6% of participants. In that study, the factors affecting dropout were training duration (4 weeks or more), training method (running), and training intensity. In addition, the HIIT method with the lowest drop-out in that study was a cycling-based intervention [16]. In addition, many preceding studies have considered the characteristics of badminton, and then selected training methods such as agility training, stepping, and full-time running to improve performance. However, this type of training cannot accurately measure exercise intensity because the heart rate response may differ from athlete to athlete even with the same training, causing the intensity of the exercise to be relative to the participant. Therefore, it is thought that training using a stationary bicycle is conducive to observing the effect of training according to absolute exercise intensity [16]. In the end, for effective HIIT, it is necessary to study the application of the exercise period or the exercise method and its effect. Therefore, in this study, we attempted to analyze the results of applying an HIIT program to adolescent badminton players for 4 weeks. For this, the HIIT performed was centered on Wingate-based training to improve anaerobic power, and routine moderate continuous training (MCT) was performed to improve muscle strength and endurance, and this was compared to HIIT. MCT is a training method traditionally applied to athletes and the public based on continuous medium-intensity exercise [17].

2. Materials and Methods

2.1. Participants

Participants were youth badminton players who visited an athlete training center. Initially, 20 middle school students and 20 high school students were recruited, but only 15 males aged 13–15 and 17 males aged 16–18 were included in this study. Excluded subjects were 5 middle school students and 3 high school students who were currently injured ($n = 2$), did not agree to participate in the study ($n = 2$), or did not complete the experiment during training ($n = 4$). Female students were excluded because there may be gender differences in the effectiveness of training. The final 32 participants did not state that they had chronic pain in the back, knees, and ankles in a questionnaire, and did not have problems with running, jumping, and cutting movements. Athletes checked the availability and safety of the program and athletes and staff were informed of the use of the training and test results for research purposes. Those who provided written consent then completed baseline testing. In a visit to the center, body composition and physical examinations were tested, followed by the Wingate anaerobic power test and an isokinetic test. The 32 participants were randomly divided into two groups: HIIT (the intervention group) and MCT (the control group), with 16 members each. A schematic diagram of the study is presented in Figure 1.

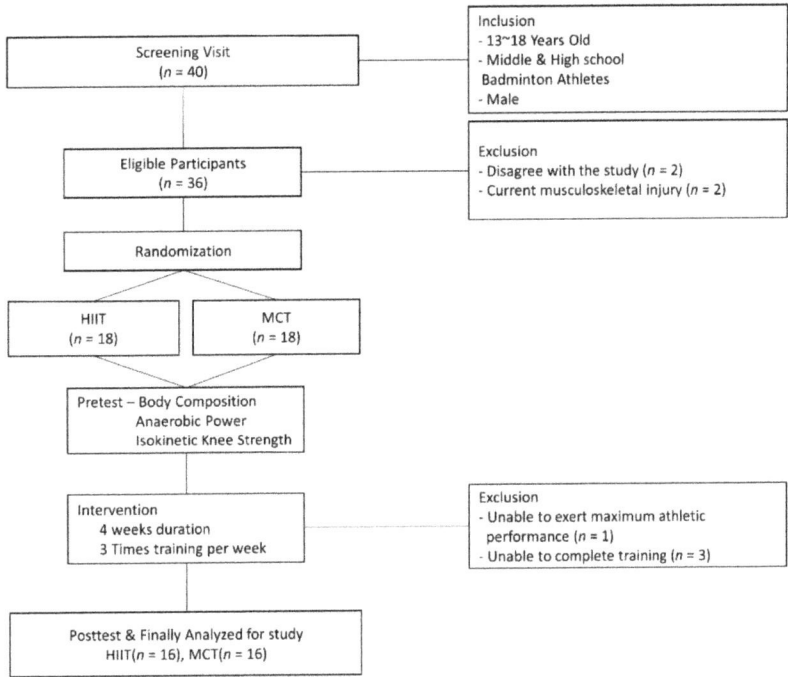

Figure 1. The design of Study; HIIT, high-intensity interval training; MCT, moderate continuous training.

2.2. Examination

2.2.1. Anthropometric Measurements

Body measurements were measured using the bioelectrical impedance method [18]. Body composition (body weight, fat mass, and muscle mass) were measured using an Inbody 770 (Biospace, Seoul, Korea) from Biospace. Body fat mass and muscle mass were each divided by body weight and converted into percentages. For an accurate examination, the hands and feet were washed with alcohol to remove sweat, and both arms and legs were abducted and measured at 30 degrees so that the armpits and the groin did not touch each other. In addition, prior to the test, the subject fasted for 8 h and either controlled or measured actions such as high-intensity exercise or sauna use, which may cause water loss. The training was conducted during the winter season (January to February), when the athletes were not in season, so body composition analysis was not affected by in-season training or playing.

2.2.2. Isokinetic Strength Test

Isokinetic muscle function was measured using a CSMi dynamometer and HUMAC software (CSMi HUMAC NORM, Stoughton, MA, USA, 2015). To increase the reliability and validity of accurate measurements and tests, the laboratory temperature was maintained at 20 °C to 25 °C, and there was no excessive eating or high-intensity exercise before the test. The extension and flexion of the knee joint were measured, an angular velocity of 60 degrees was set to measure muscle strength, and an angular velocity of 240 degrees was set to measure muscle endurance. Subjects were seated and the knee axis was aligned with the lateral epicondyle of the femur. The ankle pad was fixed to fit the distal part of the tibia. In addition, it was fixed using a pad so that the thigh and upper body did not move. The test subjects performed knee extension and flexion with concentric contraction. Sufficient explanation was given to help understand the test, and practice before the test was conducted. To induce familiarity with the test, the exercises were performed with submaximal muscle contraction 3 times at an angular velocity of 60 degrees and 3 times at a high speed at 240 degrees. The test range was set to 0–90 degrees, and the starting posture was measured at the 90-degree knee posture with the examiner's signal first, followed by flexion with the next signal. After the practice, the actual test was measured 4 times at 60°/s, and the muscle endurance was measured by repeating it 25 times at 240°/s. Muscle strength was measured based on peak torque, and the unit was a newton meter (Nm), and an absolute value and a relative value of torque per body weight were used. Muscular endurance was measured based on the total amount of work performed 25 times at an angular velocity of 240 degrees with joules as the units, and absolute and relative values were used in the same way. If there was a past injury or pain in the knee, the healthy knee was examined first. After measuring both sides, the average values of both sides were used for analysis.

2.2.3. Wingate Test

The Wingate test is a method designed to measure the anaerobic power for the load (kp; 1 kp = 50 watt) multiplied by 0.075 by weight, as suggested by Bar-Or [19]. Kp is a unit of force, and 1 kp is the magnitude of gravity for an object with a mass of 1 kg. In addition, the Wingate anaerobic test is the most commonly used method for testing the anaerobic power of athletes [20]. The Wingate test was performed using a cycle ergometer (Monark model 864 Crescent AB, Varberg, Sweden). The seat height was adjusted so that when the pedal was at the 6 o'clock position, the knee angles were 25 to 35 degrees [21,22].

The Wingate test includes 3 to 5 min of warm-up and exercise, with 80 revolutions per minute (RPM) under a light load of 50 watts (1 kp). When the participant's preparation is complete, the examiner gives a "start" signal, and the calculated load (weight × 0.075; kp) is applied at the same time. The subject tries to exert the maximum RPM for 30 s, the inspector records revolutions per minute (RPM) every 5 s, and the highest RPM, minimum RPM, and average RPM are recorded at the end of the test. The maximum power was calculated throughout the test using the following formula.

$$\text{Peak Power} = \text{Peak RPM}/12 \times \text{kp} \times 6/0.083/6.12; \text{ (unit: watt)}$$

In addition, the peak power was corrected to calculate the peak power per body weight (Peak Power/weight; watt) and the fatigue index (peak RPM − Lowest RPM/peak RPM × 100; %) was measured. After one test, a 2-min rest period was given. During this time, the pedal did not stop and 80 RPM at 1 kp was maintained. The test was repeated and measured five times in total.

2.3. Training Programs

2.3.1. High-Intensity Interval Training (HIIT)

HIIT is based on the training theory recommended by the American College of Sports Medicine (ACSM) [23], and this study used the same repeated Wingate efforts method used in Takei's study [24]. The purpose of anaerobic training is to strengthen the ability to move quickly, start quickly, exercise in a short amount of time, and sustain the high-intensity exercise necessary for badminton games. Due to the nature of badminton, one rally (the game time for which the score is recorded) is about 12 s on average; training under an extreme load for 30 s is designed to improve performance, considering that a rally often lasts up to 30 s [25]. The exercise program in this study was carried out using a stationary bicycle. The athletes trained three times a week. The warm-up and cool-down periods involved cycling at a low intensity for 5–10 min and 40–50%, respectively. A warm-up was performed while applying a load of 1 kp and maintaining a speed of 80 RPM. When the heart rate exceeded 50% of the maximum heart rate, the load was lowered or the RPM was adjusted to lower the heart rate. The total exercise period was 30 min. The exercise portion included a total of 10 bouts and was performed with an intensity of 90% heart rate maximum (HRmax) or higher for 30 s per 1 bout. The break time given per bout was 150 s, but during this break, exercise was maintained at a 50% HRmax level. The heart rate

(Polar RS400, USA) was continuously checked, and if the subject's heart rate dropped or the participant was tired, they were verbally encouraged. To improve anaerobic power, training was conducted to operate the pedal as quickly as possible at a given load for 30 s at 1 bout. Details on training are shown in Table 1.

Table 1. Specific program of High-Intensity Interval Training (HIIT).

Frequency and Duration	Time		Program	Intensity
	5~10 min		Warm-up	40~50% HRmax, 50 RPM
3 times/week For 4 weeks Training	30 min/day	30 s	1st bout	Beyond 90% HRmax, Maximal Effort
		150 s	rest	Maintain 50% HRmax, 80 RPM
		30 s	2nd bout	Beyond 90% HRmax, Maximal Effort
		150 s	rest	Maintain 50% HRmax, 80 RPM
		30 s	3th bout	Beyond 90% HRmax, Maximal Effort
		150 s	rest	Maintain 50% HRmax, 80 RPM
		30 s	4th bout	Beyond 90% HRmax, Maximal Effort
		150 s	rest	Maintain 50% HRmax, 80 RPM
		30 s	5th bout	Beyond 90% HRmax, Maximal Effort
		150 s	rest	Maintain 50% HRmax, 80 RPM
		30 s	6th bout	Beyond 90% HRmax, Maximal Effort
		150 s	rest	Maintain 50% HRmax, 80 RPM
		30 s	7th bout	Beyond 90% HRmax, Maximal Effort
		150 s	rest	Maintain 50% HRmax, 80 RPM
		30 s	8th bout	Beyond 90% HRmax, Maximal Effort
		150 s	rest	Maintain 50% HRmax, 80 RPM
		30 s	9th bout	Beyond 90% HRmax, Maximal Effort
		150 s	rest	Maintain 50% HRmax, 80 RPM
		30 s	10th bout	Beyond 90% HRmax, Maximal Effort
		150 s	rest	Maintain 50% HRmax, 80 RPM
	5~10 min		Clean-up	40~50% HRmax, 50 RPM

Abbreviation: RPM, revolutions per minute; HRmax, heart rate maximum.

2.3.2. Moderate Continuous Training (MCT)

MCT refers to a general training method for muscle strength and endurance and consists of an exercise program with a total of 12 bouts. According to the training method recommended by ACSM, it includes warm-up exercises for 5–10 min, the main exercise for 30 min, and a cool-down exercise for 5–10 min [23]. The MCT group completed the same warm-ups as the HIIT group. In the main exercise section, the upper and lower body were trained with 6 types of exercises each. Weight training for muscle strength was set to 80–85% of 1 repetition maximum (RM) and 3 sets of 10 were performed. Exercise for muscular endurance was 1 RM. Participants trained in 3 sets of 25 reps by setting a 50–60% intensity of 1 RM. The equipment used in the main exercise session used 6 types of lower body exercise machines (leg extension, leg curl, leg press, inner thigh, hip abduction, and total hip extension) and upper body machines (abdominal, rotary torso, shoulder press, and chest press, lat-pulldown, and long pull). One bout consisted of 3 sets, and each set was performed 10 times to increase muscle strength and 25 times to increase endurance. The rest time was 30 s per set and 1 min per bout. During the total 4-week training period, in the 1st and 3rd weeks, the focus was on increasing muscle strength, and in the 2nd and 4th weeks, the focus was on increasing muscle endurance. Details on training are shown in Table 2.

Table 2. Specific programs of Moderate Continuous Training (MCT).

Frequency and Duration		Time and Method		Program	Intensity
		5~10 min		Warm-up	Cycle, 50 watt, 60~70 RPM
3 times/week For 4 weeks Training	30 min	Upper Extremity, 6 bouts, Lower Extremity, 6 bouts Total: 12 bouts 10 repetitions × 3 sets (for strength), 25 repetition × 3 sets (for endurance) Rest per set: 30 s Rest per bout: 60 s	Lower Extremity	Leg Extension Leg Curl Leg Press Inner Thigh Outer Thigh Total Hip Extension	10 repetitions × 3 sets (for strength), 1 RM 80%~85%, 25 repetition × 3 sets (for endurance) 1 RM 50%~60% 1st, 3rd weeks: Strength training 2nd, 4th weeks: Endurance training
			Upper Extremity	Abdominal Rotary Torso Shoulder Press Chest Press Lat-Pulldown Back Extension	
		5~10 min		Clean-up	Cycle, 50 watt, 60~70 RPM

RPM, revolutions per minute; HR, heart rate; RM, repetition maximum.

2.3.3. Data Analysis

Data were analyzed using SPSS 25.0 (IBM SPSS Ltd., Chicago, IL, USA) and were recorded as mean and standard deviation. The nonparametric method was applied, and the paired *t*-test was performed using the Wilcoxon method for the before and after comparison by means of repeated intra-group measurements, and the independent *t*-test was performed using the Mann–Whitney method for comparisons between the two groups. Repeated two-way ANOVA was performed to analyze the differences between time and group and before and after training. The significance level was set to $p < 0.05$.

3. Results

3.1. Participants' Characteristics

Table 3 describes the general characteristics of the participants. There was no significant difference between the groups in the age, height, weight, and body mass index (BMI) values of the HIIT group and the MCT group.

Table 3. General characteristics of participants.

Variables	HIIT	MCT	p
Age, years	16.3 ± 1.2	16.5 ± 1.0	0.213
Height, cm	174.9 ± 3.5	175.7 ± 3.1	0.512
Weight, kg	65.1 ± 6.8	66.0 ± 5.4	0.631
BMI, kg/m^2	21.5 ± 1.8	21.7 ± 1.5	0.418

HIIT, high-intensity interval training; MCT, moderate continuous training, BMI, body mass index.

3.2. Body Fat and Muscle Changes before and after Training

Table 4 shows the changes in fat and muscle after the 4-week training in the HIIT group and the MCT group. There was no statistical difference between groups before training in all items. In the HIIT group, body fat and body fat percentage decreased statistically significantly after training. There was also a significant decrease between groups. However, there was no statistical significance in terms of the muscle mass and muscle ratio after training in either group. In the MCT group, there was no statistically significant difference in any items before and after training.

Table 4. Changes in body composition between groups according to training.

Variables	Group	Pre	Post	Diff (%)	Pre–Post, p	Time * Group, p
Fat, kg	HIIT	7.2 ± 2.2	6.6 ± 2.2	−9.1	0.016*	0.019 *
	MCT	7.4 ± 1.9	6.9 ± 1.7	−7.2	0.221	
	p	0.125	0.021 *			
Fat, %	HIIT	11.1 ± 2.6	10.2 ± 2.6	−7.8	0.022 *	0.028 *
	MCT	11.2 ± 2.7	10.5 ± 2.4	−6.8	0.191	
	p	0.214	0.043 *			
Muscle, kg	HIIT	30.8 ± 3.2	31.4 ± 3.4	1.9	0.121	0.415
	MCT	31.2 ± 2.8	31.6 ± 2.7	1.3	0.164	
	p	0.119	0.213			
Muscle, %	HIIT	47.3 ± 1.4	48.8 ± 2.0	3.1	0.144	0.612
	MCT	47.2 ± 1.5	48.1 ± 1.4	1.7	0.109	
	p	0.258	0.121			

* $p < 0.05$; HIIT, high-intensity interval training; MCT, moderate continuous training; Diff, different between pre- and post-training.

3.3. Change in Anaerobic Power

Table 5 shows the results of anaerobic power, determined through the Wingate test. A total of five sets of Wingate tests were performed, and peak power and fatigue index were displayed according to the weight of each set. As a result, in the case of peak power, there was no statistical difference between the anaerobic power test and the fatigue index test performed before training in both the HIIT group and the MCT group. After 4 weeks of training, there was a statistically significant improvement in peak power and fatigue index in sets 1 and 2 in both groups. However, in the case of the HIIT group, statistically significant improvements in peak power and fatigue index were observed in the anaerobic power tests of three and four sets. In the case of the MCT group, the peak power and fatigue index were not different from the pre-test values in the 3rd and 4th sets. In the case of the 5th set, the peak power did not change in both groups, but the fatigue index had a statistically significant effect in the HIIT group.

Table 5. Anaerobic power testing with the Wingate ergometer test.

Variables	Group	Pre	Post	Diff (%)	Pre–Post, p	Time * Group, p
Peak Power (P.P./BW)						
1	HIIT	11.3 ± 1.4	12.9 ± 1.8	12.4	0.003 *	0.314
	MCT	11.6 ± 1.4	12.4 ± 1.2	6.5	0.004 *	
	p	0.524	0.129			
2	HIIT	11.2 ± 1.5	12.3 ± 1.5	8.9	0.007 *	0.546
	MCT	11.4 ± 2.3	12.1 ± 1.1	5.8	0.019 *	
	p	0.268	0.211			
3	HIIT	10.9 ± 1.7	11.8 ± 1.4	6.8	0.029 *	0.019 *
	MCT	10.8 ± 1.6	11.4 ± 1.0	5.3	0.121	
	p	0.645	0.014 *			
4	HIIT	10.1 ± 1.2	11.0 ± 1.9	7.3	0.012 *	0.021 *
	MCT	10.2 ± 1.4	10.5 ± 2.1	2.9	0.062	
	p	0.341	0.011 *			
5	HIIT	9.3 ± 1.8	9.5 ± 1.7	2.1	0.445	0.129
	MCT	9.1 ± 1.6	9.3 ± 4.8	2.2	0.741	
	p	0.412	0.064			
Fatigue Index (F.I.)						
1	HIIT	32.4 ± 9.9	26.8 ± 10.6	−20.9	<0.001 *	0.841
	MCT	35.2 ± 10.9	28.5 ± 12.5	−23.5	0.003 *	
	p	0.512	0.721			

Table 5. Cont.

Variables	Group	Pre	Post	Diff (%)	Pre–Post, p	Time * Group, p
2	HIIT	40.3 ± 9.6	31.3 ± 10.1	−28.8	0.003 *	0.743
	MCT	42.7 ± 10.5	34.3 ± 14.9	−24.5	0.014 *	
	p	0.218	0.119			
3	HIIT	45.5 ± 9.2	39.0 ± 10.8	−16.7	0.029 *	0.032 *
	MCT	47.5 ± 11.3	45.0 ± 13.4	−5.6	0.121	
	p	0.347	0.024 *			
4	HIIT	49.4 ± 14.2	42.7 ± 12.5	−15.7	0.012 *	0.017 *
	MCT	50.0 ± 9.3	47.4 ± 13.9	−5.5	0.062	
	p	0.419	0.022 *			
5	HIIT	54.0 ± 15.0	51.0 ± 11.8	−5.9	0.045 *	0.003 *
	MCT	55.9 ± 12.9	54.4 ± 16.8	−2.8	0.741	
	p	0.612	0.019 *			

* $p < 0.05$; HIIT, high-intensity interval training; MCT, moderate continuous training; Diff, different between pre- and post-testing; P.P., peak power; BW, body weight; F.I., fatigue index.

3.4. Heart Rate Change after Anaerobic Power Test

Table 6 shows the pre-post results in regard to heart rate after the Wingate test. The heart rate at 1 min after the end of the test was subtracted from the maximum heart rate found through each set, and the value was divided by the maximum heart rate and expressed as a percentage. There was no statistical change in either group.

Table 6. Heart rate after the Wingate test.

Set	Group	Pre	Post	Diff (%)	Pre–Post, p	Time * Group, p
1	HIIT	39.3 ± 4.5	42.0 ± 3.1	6.4	0.412	0.211
	MCT	41.0 ± 3.6	43.4 ± 4.1	5.5	0.319	
	p	0.514	0.748			
2	HIIT	35.3 ± 6.7	38.2 ± 4.5	7.6	0.424	0.342
	MCT	37.5 ± 2.5	41.8 ± 5.8	10.3	0.511	
	p	0.126	0.419			
3	HIIT	30.2 ± 5.1	33.0 ± 7.4	8.5	0.671	0.417
	MCT	32.5 ± 4.8	31.2 ± 4.7	−4.2	0.546	
	p	0.513	0.641			
4	HIIT	20.2 ± 6.6	24.2 ± 4.3	16.5	0.541	0.784
	MCT	19.9 ± 6.9	23.4 ± 5.9	15.0	0.097	
	p	0.663	0.518			
5	HIIT	19.3 ± 7.2	19.6 ± 5.8	1.5	0.417	0.646
	MCT	18.6 ± 8.5	21.6 ± 6.9	13.9	0.211	
	p	0.248	0.820			

Heart rate = ((max − recovery 1 min)/max) × 100; HIIT, high-intensity interval training; MCT, moderate continuous training; Diff, different between pre- and post-testing.

3.5. Isokinetic Muscle Function

Table 7 shows the pre-post results for the isokinetic muscle function test. In both the HIIT and MCT groups, there was no statistically significant difference between the groups in the pre-test period before training at an angular velocity of 60 degrees and an angular velocity of 240 degrees. After 4 weeks of training, there was a statistically significant increase in extension, extension/kg, flexion, and flexion/kg in both groups at a low speed of 60 degrees. However, there was no difference between the groups. However, in the high-speed test at 240 degrees, there was a statistically significant change before and after testing only in the HIIT group.

Table 7. Isokinetic strength test.

Variables	Group	Pre	Post	Diff (%)	Pre–Post, p	Time * Group, p
60°/s, Ext, Nm	HIIT	194.9 ± 30.4	223.4 ± 31.6	12.8	0.010 *	0.122
	MCT	201.9 ± 33.7	212.5 ± 28.3	5.0	0.015 *	
	p	0.121	0.221			
60°/s, Ext, Nm/kg	HIIT	2.99 ± 0.31	3.43 ± 0.31	13.1	0.011 *	0.746
	MCT	3.05 ± 0.42	3.22 ± 0.36	5.0	0.003 *	
	p	0.515	0.153			
60°/s, Flx, Nm	HIIT	117.8 ± 17.2	132.2 ± 13.9	10.9	0.002 *	0.879
	MCT	122.6 ± 24.5	129.2 ± 17.7	5.1	0.004 *	
	p	0.247	0.412			
60°/s, Flx, Nm/kg	HIIT	1.81 ± 0.26	2.03 ± 0.26	11.3	0.045 *	0.412
	MCT	1.86 ± 0.31	1.96 ± 0.21	5.1	0.014 *	
	p	0.416	0.163			
240°/s, Ext, total joule	HIIT	2690.4 ± 540.9	2900.9 ± 561.7	7.2	0.003 *	0.035 *
	MCT	2609.4 ± 447.1	2763.9 ± 456.5	5.6	0.015 *	
	p	0.258	0.011 *			
240°/s, Ext, Total Joule/kg	HIIT	41.32 ± 6.04	44.56 ± 5.81	7.3	0.005 *	0.002 *
	MCT	39.53 ± 6.60	41.86 ± 7.12	5.5	0.129	
	p	0.426	0.035 *			
240°/s, Flx, total Joule	HIIT	1576.7 ± 281.5	1899.8 ± 318.4	17.0	0.006 *	0.004 *
	MCT	1608.8 ± 336.2	1767.8 ± 309.7	9.0	0.217	
	p	0.416	0.003 *			
240°/s, Flx, total Joule/kg	HIIT	24.21 ± 3.94	29.17 ± 3.33	17.0	0.002 *	0.005 *
	MCT	24.37 ± 5.19	26.82 ± 4.34	9.1	0.059	
	p	0.641	0.012 *			

* $p < 0.05$; HIIT, high-intensity interval training; MCT, moderate continuous training; Diff, different between pre- and post-testing.

4. Discussion

There are several studies that have applied HIIT to badminton players. In a study conducted by Wee, 18 college badminton players underwent HIIT training for 4 weeks; their improvement in mean power was statistically significant in relation to VO2 max and anaerobic power ability [26]. Samsir reported a statistically significant increase in VO2 max and a 20-m shuttle run test, which is a comprehensive test of anaerobic ability, agility, and muscular endurance after HIIT for 10 weeks in 16 male adolescent badminton players [27]. Badminton requires better stamina than other sports [28]; based on this, this study also examined badminton players, and HIIT showed a statistically significant improvement in terms of body fat, anaerobic power, and isokinetic muscle endurance compared to MCT.

There are many studies that relate to the training period. In the case of short-term training, an improvement in physical strength and performance was reported even after 4–6 weeks of training [29]. In addition, Pritchard's results showed that after the general population used HIIT 3 days a week for 4 weeks, the isometric strength of the lower body when using a leg extension machine, the isometric strength of the upper body when using a chest press machine, and standing jump performance increased statistically significantly [30]. In this study, the body fat, anaerobic ability, fatigue, and muscle endurance among the isokinetic muscle functions of the HIIT group improved in only a short period of 4 weeks. For the MCT group, there was no change in body composition, but the first two sets showed a significant increase in anaerobic power and a statistically significant decrease in muscle fatigue from the pre-test period. In addition, knee extension muscle strength and muscle endurance using isokinetic equipment showed a statistically significant increase in both HIIT and MCT groups compared to the pre-test period. Regarding knee flexion, the HIIT group showed a statistically significant increase in both muscle strength and muscle endurance. In the MCT group, there was a statistically significant increase in muscle strength, but the improvement in muscle endurance was not statistically significant.

Four weeks of HIIT proved to be an important factor in demonstrating the effectiveness of short-term training in fat and muscle changes in athletes. However, opinions are divided on the clear training effect of HIIT for youth. After reviewing the effect of short-term HIIT training as reported in 13 studies, Eddolls observed that six studies reported statistically significant changes in body mass index (BMI), %Fat, and fat-free mass (FFM) [31]. However, there was no consensus even on this result. Eddolls's review showed some studies that reported increased BMI, and others that reported increased FFM. In this study, after training, the HIIT group showed a statistically significant loss of body fat. This should highlight how HIIT is based on aerobic exercise, whereas MCT is based on unilateral strength training and therefore the principle of training specificity [32]. Schubert reported that the resting metabolic rate (RMR) and VO2 max increased statistically significantly and body fat decreased due to Wingate training in 30 men and women who were not athletes over 4 weeks [33]. Therefore, it has been reported that Wingate-based training can have a significant beneficia; effect within a four-week training period.

There have been several prior studies on anaerobic power. According to Forster, the peak power output increased by 18% as a result of HIIT training for 55 healthy college students conducted three times a week for 8 weeks [34]. In this study, anaerobic power was increased in both HIIT and MCT groups even during the short training period of 4 weeks. A total of five sets of anaerobic power were tested. In particular, the HIIT group showed an increase of 12.4% in the first set, which was statistically significant up to the fourth set. In the case of the MCT group, there was a statistically significant increase in sets 1 and 2 compared to the pre-test period, but not in sets 3–5. As the set was repeated, the anaerobic power and muscular endurance of badminton players decreased, but the HIIT group was able to maintain the expression of power after 4 weeks of training, which is expected to improve performance. Similarly, muscle fatigue can be predicted based on the correlation between the highest and lowest RPMs during the test. In this area, the HIIT group showed a statistically significant decrease in fatigue compared to the MCT group. In the MCT group, after 4 weeks of training, there was a statistically significant decrease in the 1st and 2nd sets, but there was no significant difference from the pre-test period in the 3rd and 5th sets. Anaerobic power means instantaneous explosive power, and fatigue refers to how well it can be maintained at the highest RPM. Badminton rallies last up to 30 s, so fatigue and muscular endurance are important for players.

After the anaerobic power test, the heart rate indicates the body's physiological response. In this study, there was no statistically significant change after training in both HIIT and MCT groups. Ramos et al. studied the effect of HIIT and MCT training on vascular function using a meta-analysis method and concluded that HIIT had a significant effect of 2.26% ($p < 0.05$) on vascular function, such as brachial artery flow-mediated dilation (FMD), compared to MCT, which in turn had a positive effect on biomarkers related to cardiorespiratory fitness and vascular function [35]. The ability to recover heart rate after an extreme anaerobic power test is also included in vascular function. However, there was no change in heart rate after training in this study. It may be that the 4-week training period was insufficient to show functional changes in heart rate. Furthermore, all of the variables that had an effect in Ramos' study involved training for at least 12 weeks. Therefore, the variables related to the heart are not likely to change with only four weeks of training. Therefore, longer-term training is necessary in future studies.

The muscle strength and endurance in this study were measured using an isokinetic device. High-intensity interval training improves the molecular signaling pathways that control changes in muscles caused by endurance training, such as mitochondrial production and the ability to transport and oxidize carbohydrates and fats [36]. In this study, an angular velocity of 60°/s and an angular velocity of 240°/s were measured, and the measurement items were measured strength and endurance, respectively. As a result of 4-week training, there was a statistically significant improvement in muscle strength in both the HIIT and MCT groups, and no improvement in muscle endurance was observed in the MCT group. There was no statistical difference between groups in terms of muscle strength, but the HIIT group showed more improvement than the MCT group. In muscle endurance, the HIIT group showed a statistically significant difference, whereas the MCT group did not. This implies that adaptation due to training is possible in just 4 weeks.

This study has several limitations. First, the effectiveness of training was not identified by further subdividing the age of the adolescents. Therefore, it is necessary to investigate the effect of training on badminton players in middle and high school students separately. Second, it was not possible to control for food intake or daily life activities, which may have affected the results. Third, it was not possible to conduct additional types of training and comparative analysis to determine the effect of HIIT. Therefore, further research is needed to improve these limitations.

5. Conclusions

The HIIT group showed decreased body fat, improved anaerobic power, improved fatigue index, knee extension and flexion muscle endurance. Therefore, it is valuable to apply a short training period of HIIT to improve performance in youth badminton players.

Author Contributions: Conceptualization, D.-H.K. and Y.-C.C.; methodology, D.-H.K.; formal analysis, Y.-C.C. and D.-S.L.; investigation, D.-H.K.; writing—original draft preparation, D.-H.K. and Y.-C.C.; writing—review and editing, D.-S.L.; supervision, Y.-C.C. and D.-S.L. All authors have read and agreed to the published version of the manuscript.

Funding: There was no support or funding from any individual or organization to conduct this study.

Institutional Review Board Statement: The study was conducted according to the guidelines of the Declaration of Helsinki, and approved by the Institutional Review Board of Gangeung-Wonju National University (2021-11).

Informed Consent Statement: Informed consent was obtained from all subjects involved in the study, and written informed consent has been obtained from the participants to publish this paper.

Data Availability Statement: The data are not publicly available due to privacy or ethical reasons.

Conflicts of Interest: The authors declare that there are no potential conflicts of interest with respect to the research, authorship, and/or publication of this article.

References

1. Seth, B. Determination factors of badminton game performance. *Int. J. Phys. Educ. Sports Health* **2016**, *3*, 20–22.
2. Zhang, Z.; Li, S.; Wan, B.; Visentin, P.; Jiang, Q.; Dyck, M.; Li, H.; Shan, G. The influence of X-factor (trunk rotation) and experience on the quality of the badminton forehand smash. *J. Hum. Kinet.* **2016**, *53*, 9–22. [CrossRef] [PubMed]
3. Raman, D.; Nageswaran, A. Effect of game-specific strength training on selected physiological variables among badminton players. *Int. J. Sci. Res.* **2013**, *1*, 1–2. [CrossRef]
4. Phomsoupha, M.; Laffaye, G. The science of badminton: Game characteristics, anthropometry, physiology, visual fitness and biomechanics. *J. Sports Med.* **2015**, *45*, 473–495. [CrossRef]
5. Van Lieshout, K.A.; Lombard, A.J. Fitness profile of elite junior South African badminton players. *Afr. J. Phys. Act. Health Sci.* **2003**, *9*, 114–120. [CrossRef]
6. Andersen, L.L.; Larsson, B.; Overgaard, H.; Aagaard, P. Torque–velocity characteristics and contractile rate of force development in elite badminton players. *J. Eur. J. Sport Sci.* **2007**, *7*, 127–134. [CrossRef]
7. Cabello, D.; Padial, P.; Lees, A.; Rivas, F. Temporal and Physiological Characteristics of Elite Women's and Men's Singles Badminton. *Int. J. Appl. Sports Sci.* **2004**, *16*, 1–12.
8. Naimo, M.; De Souza, E.; Wilson, J.; Carpenter, A.; Gilchrist, P.; Lowery, R.; Averbuch, B.; White, T.; Joy, J. High-intensity interval training has positive effects on performance in ice hockey players. *Int. J. Sports Med.* **2015**, *36*, 61–66. [CrossRef] [PubMed]
9. Kong, Z.; Fan, X.; Sun, S.; Song, L.; Shi, Q.; Nie, J. Comparison of high-intensity interval training and moderate-to-vigorous continuous training for cardiometabolic health and exercise enjoyment in obese young women: A randomized controlled trial. *PLoS ONE* **2016**, *11*, 8589. [CrossRef] [PubMed]
10. Ross, L.M.; Porter, R.R.; Durstine, J.L. High-intensity interval training (HIIT) for patients with chronic diseases. *J. Sport Health Sci.* **2016**, *5*, 139–144. [CrossRef] [PubMed]
11. Armas, C.; Kowalsky, R.J.; Hearon, C.M. Comparison of Acute Cardiometabolic Responses in a 7-Minute Body Weight Circuit to 7 Minute HIIT Training Protocol. *J. Int. J. Exerc. Sci.* **2020**, *13*, 395–409.

12. Jakovljevic, B.; Turnic, T.N.; Jeremic, N.; Jeremic, J.; Bradic, J.; Ravic, M.; Jakovljevic, V.L.; Jelic, D.; Radovanovic, D.; Pechanova, O. The impact of aerobic and anaerobic training regimes on blood pressure in normotensive and hypertensive rats: Focus on redox changes. *J. Mol. Cell. Biochem.* **2019**, *454*, 111–121. [CrossRef] [PubMed]
13. Holloway, K.; Roche, D.; Angell, P. Evaluating the progressive cardiovascular health benefits of short-term high-intensity interval training. *Eur. J. Appl. Physiol.* **2018**, *118*, 2259–2268. [CrossRef] [PubMed]
14. Klonizakis, M.; Moss, J.; Gilbert, S.; Broom, D.; Foster, J.; Tew, G.A. Low-volume high-intensity interval training rapidly improves cardiopulmonary function in postmenopausal women. *J. Menopause* **2014**, *21*, 1099–1105. [CrossRef] [PubMed]
15. Jelleyman, C.; Yates, T.; O'Donovan, G.; Gray, L.J.; King, J.A.; Khunti, K.; Davies, M.J. The effects of high-intensity interval training on glucose regulation and insulin resistance: A meta-analysis. *J. Obes. Rev.* **2015**, *16*, 942–961. [CrossRef]
16. Reljic, D.; Lampe, D.; Wolf, F.; Zopf, Y.; Herrmann, H.J.; Fischer, J. Prevalence and predictors of dropout from high-intensity interval training in sedentary individuals: A meta-analysis. *Scand. J. Med. Sci. Sports* **2019**, *29*, 1288–1304. [CrossRef]
17. Mueller, S.; Winzer, E.B.; Duvinage, A.; Gevaert, A.B.; Edelmann, F.; Haller, B.; Pieske-Kraigher, E.; Beckers, P.; Bobenko, A.; Hommel, J. Effect of High-Intensity Interval Training, Moderate Continuous Training, or Guideline-Based Physical Activity Advice on Peak Oxygen Consumption in Patients with Heart Failure with Preserved Ejection Fraction: A Randomized Clinical Trial. *J. Am. Med. Assoc.* **2021**, *325*, 542–551. [CrossRef]
18. Cornish, B. Bioimpedance analysis: Scientific background. *J. Lymphat. Res. Biol.* **2006**, *4*, 47–50. [CrossRef]
19. Bar-Or, O. The Wingate anaerobic test an update on methodology, reliability and validity. *Sports Med.* **1987**, *4*, 381–394. [CrossRef]
20. Jakovljević, D.K.; Eric, M.; Jovanovic, G.; Dimitric, G.; Cupic, M.B.; Ponorac, N. Explosive muscle power assessment in elite athletes using wingate anaerobic test. *Revista Brasileira de Medicina do Esporte* **2018**, *24*, 107–111. [CrossRef]
21. Peveler, W.W.; Pounders, J.D.; Bishop, P.A. Effects of saddle height on anaerobic power production in cycling. *J. Strength Cond. Res.* **2007**, *21*, 1023. [PubMed]
22. Moura, B.M.d.; Moro, V.L.; Rossato, M.; Lucas, R.D.d.; Diefenthaeler, F. Effects of saddle height on performance and muscular activity during the Wingate test. *J. Phys. Educ.* **2017**, *28*. [CrossRef]
23. Liguori, G. *ACSM's Guidelines for Exercise Testing and Prescription*; American College of Sports Medicine: Indianapolis, IN, USA, 2020.
24. Takei, N.; Kakinoki, K.; Girard, O.; Hatta, H. Short-Term Repeated Wingate Training in Hypoxia and Normoxia in Sprinters. *Front Sports Act. Living* **2020**, *2*, 1–8. [CrossRef] [PubMed]
25. Duncan, M.J.; Chan, C.K.; Clarke, N.D.; Cox, M.; Smith, M. The effect of badminton-specific exercise on badminton short-serve performance in competition and practice climates. *Eur. J. Sport Sci.* **2017**, *17*, 119–126. [CrossRef]
26. Wee, E.H.; Low, J.Y.; Chan, K.Q.; Ler, H.Y. Effects of High Intensity Intermittent Badminton Multi-Shuttle Feeding Training on Aerobic and Anaerobic Capacity, Leg Strength Qualities and Agility. In Proceedings of the 5th International Congress on Sport Sciences Research and Technology Support (icSPORTS 2017), Madeira, Portugal, 30–31 October 2017; Springer: Berlin/Heidelberg, Germany, 2019; pp. 39–47.
27. Samsir, M.S.; Mariappan, M.; Noordin, H.; Azmi, A.M.i.B.N. The Effects of High Intensity Functional Interval Training on Selected Fitness Components Among Young Badminton Players. In *Enhancing Health and Sports Performance by Design, Proceedings of the 2019 Movement, Health & Exercise (MoHE), Kuching, Malaysia, 30 September–2 October 2019 and International Sports Science Conference (ISSC), Bangkok, Thailand, 23–25 January 2019*; Springer: Berlin/Heidelberg, Germany, 2019; pp. 42–53.
28. Singh, J.; Raza, S.; Mohammad, A. Physical characteristics and level of performance in badminton: A relationship study. *J. Educ. Pract.* **2011**, *2*, 6–10.
29. Váczi, M.; Tollár, J.; Meszler, B.; Juhász, I.; Karsai, I. Short-term high intensity plyometric training program improves strength, power and agility in male soccer players. *J. Hum. Kinet.* **2013**, *36*, 17–26. [CrossRef]
30. Pritchard, H.J.; Barnes, M.J.; Stewart, R.J.; Keogh, J.W.; McGuigan, M.R. Short-term training cessation as a method of tapering to improve maximal strength. *J. Strength Cond. Res.* **2018**, *32*, 458–465. [CrossRef]
31. Eddolls, W.T.; McNarry, M.A.; Stratton, G.; Winn, C.O.; Mackintosh, K.A. High-intensity interval training interventions in children and adolescents: A systematic review. *J. Sports Med.* **2017**, *47*, 2363–2374. [CrossRef] [PubMed]
32. Howe, L.P.; Read, P.; Waldron, M. Muscle hypertrophy: A narrative review on training principles for increasing muscle mass. *J. Strength Cond.* **2017**, *39*, 72–81. [CrossRef]
33. Schubert, M.M.; Clarke, H.E.; Seay, R.F.; Spain, K.K. Impact of 4 weeks of interval training on resting metabolic rate, fitness, and health-related outcomes. *J. Appl. Physiol. Nutr. Metab.* **2017**, *42*, 1073–1081. [CrossRef]
34. Foster, C.; Farland, C.V.; Guidotti, F.; Harbin, M.; Roberts, B.; Schuette, J.; Tuuri, A.; Doberstein, S.T.; Porcari, J.P. The effects of high intensity interval training vs steady state training on aerobic and anaerobic capacity. *J. Sports Sci. Med.* **2015**, *14*, 747–755. [PubMed]
35. Ramos, J.S.; Dalleck, L.C.; Tjonna, A.E.; Beetham, K.S.; Coombes, J.S. The impact of high-intensity interval training versus moderate-intensity continuous training on vascular function: A systematic review and meta-analysis. *J. Sports Med.* **2015**, *45*, 679–692. [CrossRef] [PubMed]
36. MacInnis, M.J.; Gibala, M.J. Physiological adaptations to interval training and the role of exercise intensity. *J. Physiol.* **2017**, *595*, 2915–2930. [CrossRef] [PubMed]

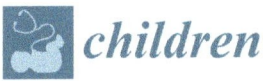

Article

Different Effects of the COVID-19 Pandemic on Exercise Indexes and Mood States Based on Sport Types, Exercise Dependency and Individual Characteristics

Alireza Aghababa [1], Georgian Badicu [2], Zahra Fathirezaie [3,*], Hadi Rohani [4], Maghsoud Nabilpour [5], Seyed Hojjat Zamani Sani [3] and Elham Khodadadeh [3]

1. Department of Sport Psychology, Sport Sciences Research Institute, Tehran 15879, Iran; alirezaaghababa@yahoo.com
2. Department of Physical Education and Special Motricity, Faculty of Physical Education and Mountain Sports, Transilvania University of Brasov, 500068 Brasov, Romania; georgian.badicu@unitbv.ro
3. Motor Behavior Faculty, Physical Education and Sport Sciences Faculty, University of Tabriz, Tabriz 51666, Iran; hojjatzamani8@gmail.com (S.H.Z.S.); khodadadehelham1995@gmail.com (E.K.)
4. Department of Exercise Physiology, Sport Sciences Research Institute, Tehran 15879, Iran; h_rohani7@yahoo.com
5. Department of Sport Physiology, Faculty of Psychology and Educational Sciences, Mohaghegh Ardabili University, Ardabil 56199, Iran; nabilpour@yahoo.com
* Correspondence: Zahra.fathirezaie@gmail.com; Tel.: +98-41-333933386

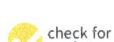

Citation: Aghababa, A.; Badicu, G.; Fathirezaie, Z.; Rohani, H.; Nabilpour, M.; Zamani Sani, S.H.; Khodadadeh, E. Different Effects of the COVID-19 Pandemic on Exercise Indexes and Mood States Based on Sport Types, Exercise Dependency and Individual Characteristics. *Children* 2021, 8, 438. https://doi.org/10.3390/children8060438

Academic Editor: Filipe Manuel Clemente

Received: 19 April 2021
Accepted: 21 May 2021
Published: 24 May 2021

Publisher's Note: MDPI stays neutral with regard to jurisdictional claims in published maps and institutional affiliations.

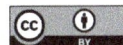

Copyright: © 2021 by the authors. Licensee MDPI, Basel, Switzerland. This article is an open access article distributed under the terms and conditions of the Creative Commons Attribution (CC BY) license (https://creativecommons.org/licenses/by/4.0/).

Abstract: Exercise indexes have been affected by the coronavirus disease 2019 (COVID-19) pandemic and its related restrictions among athletes. In the present study, we investigated the exercise frequency and intensity before and during the COVID-19 pandemic, and also current exercise dependency and mood state among non-contact individual, contact individual, and team sports athletes. A total of 1353 athletes from non-contact individual sports athletes (NCISA), contact individual sports athletes (CISA) and team sport athletes (TSA) participated; 45.4% of them were females that completed a series of self-rating questionnaires covering sociodemographic information, former and current exercise patterns, exercise dependency and mood states. NCISA had less exercise frequency than CISA, both before and during the COVID-19 pandemic, and NCISA had less exercise frequency than TSA during the COVID-19 pandemic. Regarding exercise intensity, CISA had higher scores than NCISA and TSA before the COVID-19 pandemic, and CISA had more exercise intensity than TSA during the COVID-19 pandemic. Frequency and intensity were reduced from before to during the COVID-19 pandemic in the three groups, except for TSA intensity. In addition, positive and negative mood states were correlated with exercise dependency. CISA were more discouraged and vigorous than NCISA and TSA, respectively. For NCISA, CISA, and TSA, ordinal regressions separately showed that adherence to quarantine and exercise dependency were better predictors of exercise indexes. Finally, exercise dependency subscales were different among sports, but it was not in exercise dependency itself. Although the decrease in exercise indexes was noticeable, there was no consistent pattern of change in exercise behavior in all sports. Additionally, during the COVID-19 pandemic, negative moods were predominant among all athletes. The results discussed are based on exercise nonparticipating, sport type, and affect regulation hypothesis.

Keywords: exercise indexes; exercise dependency; COVID-19 pandemic; team sports; individual sports

1. Introduction

Psychological and social pressures such as economic problems and illness may always be around us and can lead to some changes in our lifestyle [1,2]. Of course, in addition to stress, the perception of eustress can also have better effects. In fact, what we perceive from external events affects our perception, behavior, and life. The emergence of the coronavirus disease 2019 (COVID-19) is one of these stressors that has greatly affected economic, social, and even personal life. Of course, different strategies have been taken to prevent infection, and some suggestions have been made. In this regard, although the importance of maintaining exercise in all its dimensions, such as physiological or psychological effects, is recommended, the closure of sports centers and the possibility of air pollution in these spaces may have reduced the amount of physical activity (PA) during lockdown [3], and may, in turn, induce numerous health problems such as stress, depression, and anxiety related to the confinement and prolonged periods of inactivity [4]. Recent findings have shown this in various countries [5]; however, a limitation of previous studies was that apparently no distinction was made between individual and team sports athletes. For the following reason, this is critical: compared to individually exercising athletes, it is conceivable that team sports athletes decreased their exercise levels more rigorously when compared to exercise levels before the lockdown, because of social distancing. Additionally, limited training group sizes might have impacted team sports athletes more severely. Thus, the first aim of the present study was to investigate the differences in exercise frequency and intensity of individual and team sports athletes before and during the lockdown.

Decreased exercise in addition to physiologically destructive effects can also have psychological effects, although recent studies have shown a decreased PA during the COVID-19 pandemic and mood swings [6], it seems that these effects may be more in people who did collaborative in team sports compare to individual sports. Research has shown that people who do individual sports have different self-regulatory skills [7], coping strategies [8], some individual characteristics [9,10], and personality characters [11] from people who do team sports. Additionally, it has been claimed that team sport athletes are at high genetic risk of severe COVID-19 [12]. Therefore, the second aim of this study was the investigation of individual and team sport athlete's mood states during the COVID-19 pandemic. For a deeper understanding of the issue, we investigated contact and non-contract individual and team sport athletes.

In addition to the study of exercise frequency and intensity, we also predicted them by other influential factors. It seems that craving for doing a sport, which is known as exercise dependency, along with individual factors such as age and gender, are some possible predictors of exercise indexes during the COVID-19 pandemic. Therefore, the third aim of this study was predicting exercise frequency and intensity by individual characteristics including exercise dependency, age, gender, and adherence to quarantine.

Although the positive relationship between higher expert-paced PA intensity levels and mood states have been shown [13–15], it seems that lockdown-related change in PA levels is associated with mood, which, in turn, is influenced by the type of physical activity (team or individual sport) and exercise dependency in individuals. As previous studies have shown [16], there seemed to be a conceptual relationship between mood states during the COVID-19 pandemic and exercise dependency in this study; therefore, we investigated possible relationships between them among all groups.

Mental health conditions among the general and professional populations were reported by cross-sectional [17] and longitudinal [18] studies during the COVID-19 pandemic, but there currently is not clear evidence on the possible effect of the dependence of exercise on the other athlete's behavior which, in turn, could affect PA. Therefore, in this study, we investigated non-contact individual sport athletes (NCISA), contact individual sport athletes (CISA), and team sport athletes (TSA) in terms of exercise indexes, exercise dependency, and mood states.

To the best of our knowledge, no study to date has evaluated the differences in frequency and intensity of PA, exercise dependency and positive/negative mood states, and their possible differences among individual and team sport athletes during the COVID-19 pandemic. Therefore, we wanted to find out the difference in exercise characteristics and mood states among contact and non-contract individual and team sport athletes. Additionally, we investigated the possible relationship between exercise dependency and positive/negative mood states. Finally, we looked to find out whether exercise frequency and intensity could be predicted by exercise dependency, age, gender, and adherence to quarantine during the COVID-19 pandemic.

2. Materials and Methods

2.1. Procedure

Individual and team sports athletes were approached via social network sites (SNS) to participate in the present online study, and they were asked to fill out a questionnaire package on exercise frequency and intensity before and during the COVID-19 pandemic, mood states, and exercise dependency from 5 March to 30 April 2020. Before starting, the objectives of the research, the anonymous data gathering techniques, the confidential data handling practices, and the ethical approval of the study were explained to the participants on the first pages of the study. Next, participants accepted informed consent by clicking a box of agreement. Additionally, the Human Research Ethics Board at the Sport Sciences Research Institute of Iran approved the study (approval ID: IR.SSRC.REC.1399.070), which was performed in accordance with the last revision of the Declaration of Helsinki [19].

2.2. Participants

A sample of 1353 Iranian athletes with 45.4% females participated in this study. They included non-contact individual sportspeople (skating, $n = 95$; fitness and body building, $n = 165$; swimming, $n = 80$; gymnastics, $n = 70$) with athletes whose mean age was 26.8 years (SD = 10.53 years); contact individual sport athletes (karate, $n = 85$; taekwondo, $n = 87$; judo, $n = 94$, wushu, $n = 76$; boxing, $n = 91$; wrestling, $n = 68$) whose mean age was 23.76 years (SD = 9.86 years); and team sport athletes whose mean age was 24.79 years (SD = 10.41 years) (football, $n = 102$; futsal, $n = 85$; volleyball, $n = 98$; handball, $n = 115$; and basketball, $n = 110$).

2.3. Measures

2.3.1. Exercise Level

Exercise levels were measured by inquiring about the type, frequency, and intensity of exercise (from low to very high) before and during the COVID-19 pandemic, which was extracted from the 5-item PA questionnaire developed based on Cho's study [20]. The reliability and validity of this tool have been confirmed by Cho [21]. The first question was related to the type of activities in which the athletes participated before/during the COVID-19 pandemic. Individual and team sports were the main sports of athletes before the COVID-19 pandemic; an open-ended question was asked about physical activities during the COVID-19 pandemic. The second question was "before/during the COVID-19 pandemic, how often do you participate in the activity?" The choices were "every day, 6 days/week, 5 days/week, 4 days/week, 3 days/week, 2 days/week, 1 day/week and anytime". Additionally, the last question was "how intensely do you participate in the activity before/during the COVID-19 pandemic?" The choices for intensity were "light, moderate hard and very hard".

2.3.2. Mood State

To evaluate positive and negative mood states, we used a shortened version of the Brunel Mood Scale (BRUMS) [22,23]. The questionnaire included items related to 16 mood states. In the mood test, the participants were asked to express their current feelings according to the instructions. Each response was scored on a five-point scale (ranging from 0 = no to 4 = extremely). The internal consistency values (Cronbach's alpha) of all dimensions and the total scale ranged from 0.82 to 0.96 [24], while in the present study the total scale was 0.90.

2.3.3. Exercise Dependency

The Exercise Dependency measure was measured via 16 items on a seven-point Likert scale. It included the following five factors: expected positive consequences, interference with social life, health, withdrawal symptoms, and exercise as a possibility to compensate for psychological problems. This scale has already been used by previous researchers and validated with internal consistency ($\alpha = 0.643$–0.808) and fitted the model [25].

Additionally, questions regarding some individual characteristics such as age and social measures concerning the COVID-19 pandemic were asked, such as adherence to quarantine, type and duration of applied confinements, social distancing, and lockdown of gyms, outdoor sports centers and parks.

2.4. Statistical Analysis

Differences in exercise indexes among athletes of different sports were analyzed by Kruskal–Wallis one-way analysis of variance for between-group effects, and Mann–Whitney U test for within-group effects. Additionally, multivariate analysis of variance was used to investigate negative and positive mood states among different sport groups during the COVID-19 pandemic. In addition, the relationship of exercise dependency with mood states was analyzed by Spearman's correlation coefficients. Additionally, ordinal regressions were used to predicting exercise frequency and intensity by exercise dependency, age, gender, and adherence to quarantine among different sport groups. Finally, one-way analysis of variance and MANOVA were used to analyze exercise dependency and its subscales among different sport groups. The level of significance was set at alpha < 0.05. All statistical analyses were computed utilizing IBM Corp. Released 2015. IBM SPSS Statistics for Windows, Version 23.0. Armonk, NY, USA: IBM Corp and Microsoft Excel (2013).

3. Results

3.1. Descriptive Statistics of Studied Variables

Table 1 shows the mean or median scores of exercise frequency and intensity before and during the COVID-19 pandemic, as well as mood states, exercise dependency, and their subscales.

Table 1. Descriptive statistics of studied variables.

Variables		NCISA Mean/Median	CISA Mean/Median	TSA Mean/Median
Before COVID-19	Frequency	3.87	4.29	4.30
	Intensity	2.68	3.00	2.66
During COVID-19	Frequency	2.52	3.14	4.65
	Intensity	1.93	2.03	1.87
Mood state (Total score)		39.17	40.67	39.68
Positive moods		7.70	8.03	7.62
Negative moods		31.4	32.64	32.05
Exercise dependency (Total score)		66.68	67.02	64.67
Expected positive consequences		17.04	17.05	16.45
Withdrawal symptoms		13.54	14.27	13.14
Exercise as a possibility to compensate for psychological problems		11.21	11.59	11.13
Interference with social life		7.44	7.28	7.63
Health		16.75	16.14	15.70

3.2. Exercise Indexes of Different Sport Athletes

Kruskal–Wallis one-way analysis of variance showed that NCISA had less frequent exercise than CISA, both before and during the COVID-19 pandemic, and NCISA had less frequent exercise than TSA during the COVID-19 pandemic. Regarding exercise intensity, CISA had higher scores than NCISA and TSA before the COVID-19 pandemic, and CISA had higher exercise intensity than TSA during the COVID-19 pandemic (Table 2).

Table 2. Group differences of exercise frequency and intensity before and during COVID-19.

Exercise	(I)	(J)	Frequency				Intensity			
			Kruskal Wallis	p	Test Statistics	Adj. P	Kruskal Wallis	p	Test Statistics	Adj. P
Before COVID-19	NCISA	CISA	7.27	0.026 *	−65.28	0.034 *	58.71	0.0001 *	−152.53	0.000 *
	NCISA	TSA			−55.99	0.096			4.43	0.999
	CISA	TSA			9.29	0.99			156.97	0.000 *
During COVID-19	NCISA	CISA	130.86	0.000 *	−91.24	0.001 *	9.30	0.01 *	−42.08	0.216
	NCISA	TSA			−291.91	0.000 *			26.37	0.806
	CISA	TSA			−200.67	0.000 *			68.45	0.008 *

NCISA, non-contact individual sport athletes; CISA, contact individual sport athletes; TSA, team sport athletes; * $p \leq 0.05$.

In addition, Mann–Whitney U test for within-group effects showed that the frequency and intensity were reduced from before to during the COVID-19 pandemic in the three groups, except for TSA intensity (Tables 1 and 3). However, this latter variable was not significant.

Table 3. Intergroup changes in exercise frequency and intensity from before to during COVID-19.

Group	(I)	(J)	Frequency		Intensity	
			Wilcoxon Statistics	p	Wilcoxon Statistics	p
NCISA	Before COVID-19	During COVID-19	8275.50	0.000 *	2051.00	0.000 *
CISA	Before COVID-19	During COVID-19	13,884	0.000 *	2128.50	0.000 *
TSA	Before COVID-19	During COVID-19	32,120	0.0052	3228.00	0.000 *

NCISA, non-contact individual sport athletes; CISA, contact individual sport athletes; TSA, team sport athletes; * $p \leq 0.05$.

3.3. Mood States of Athletes during the COVID-19 Pandemic

Descriptive analyses of mood states (12 items for negative mood states and 4 items for positive mood states) among NCISA, CISA, and TSA are shown in Figure 1.

MANOVA showed that there were significant differences in negative mood states among different athletes (F = 1.66, p = 0.022, Wilks' Lambda = 0.968, Partial Eta Squared = 0.016). Thus, the pairwise comparisons showed that CISA were more discouraged than NCISA (mean differences = 0.253, p = 0.010). Additionally, positive mood state analysis showed that there were significant differences among different sports (F = 2.10, p = 0.032, Wilks' Lambda = 0.986, Partial Eta Squared = 0.007). The results showed that CISA were more vigorous than TSA (mean differences = 0.243, p = 0.005). However, there were no significant differences among other negative or positive mood states (all p-values > 0.05).

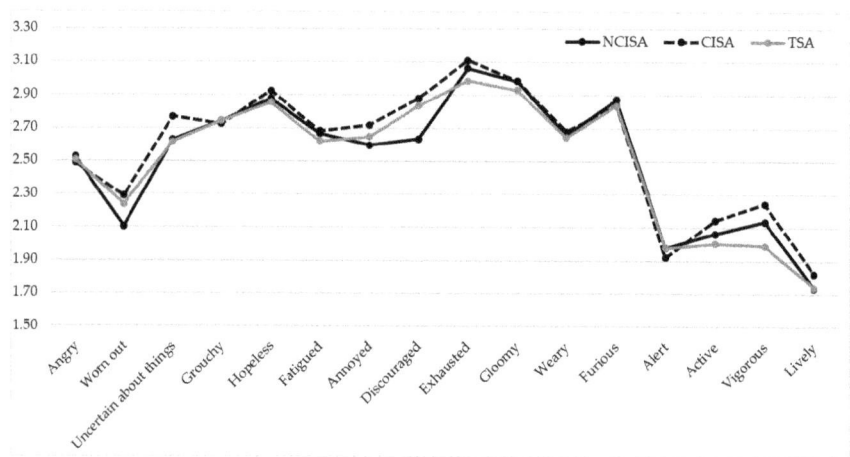

Figure 1. Mood states of different groups of athletes during the COVID-19 pandemic.

3.4. Correlation Coefficients of Exercise Dependency, Negative and Positive Mood States

The Pearson's correlation coefficients also showed that there was a positive significant relationship between exercise dependency with positive mood states (r = 0.198, p = 0.0001) and a negative significant correlation with negative mood states (r = −0.077, p = 0.008), but their effect size was very small (4% and 0.5%, respectively).

3.5. Predicting of Exercise Indexes by Exercise Dependency, Age, Gender, and Adherence to Quarantine in Different Sport Groups

Additionally, we investigated whether exercise frequency and intensity could be predicted by exercise dependency, age, gender, and adherence to quarantine among different sports. For NCISA, CISA, and TSA, ordinal regressions showed that adherence to quarantine and exercise dependency were the best predictors. (Table 4).

Table 4. Ordinal regression parameters of NCISA, CISA, and TSA during the COVID-19 pandemic.

	Sport Type	Model Fit			Goodness-of-Fit		
		−2 Log Likelihood	Chi-Squared	p	Pearson's Chi-Squared	p	Pseudo R-Square
Frequency	NCISA	1274.11	189.63	0.000 *	3087.41	0.000 *	0.41
	CISA	1497.14	168.77	0.005 *	5129.439	0.000 *	0.34
	TSA	1446.91	184.21	0.000 *	3266.846	0.015 *	0.36
Intensity	NCISA	505.69	255.54	0.000 *	936.560	0.005 *	0.58
	CISA	678.490	234.07	0.000 *	1361.711	0.000 *	0.48
	TSA	650.81	174.51	0.001 *	1057.76	0.226	0.40

NCISA, non-contact individual sport athletes; CISA, contact individual sport athletes; TSA, team sport athletes; * p ≤ 0.05.

Parameter estimates showed that exercise frequency could be predicted by exercise dependency (in the NCISA and CISA), adherence to quarantine (in the CISA and TSA), and age (in the CISA). In addition, exercise intensity could be predicted by exercise dependency (CISA), adherence to quarantine (in the NCISA and CISA), and gender (in the CISA).

3.6. Perceived Exercise Dependency and Its Subscales among Sports Groups during COVID-19

Finally, one-way analysis of variance showed that there was no significant difference in exercise dependency (total score) among different sport groups (F = 2.08, p = 0.132).

However, MANOVA (Wilk's Lambda value = 0.978, F = 2.64, p = 0.003) showed that CISA had more withdrawal symptoms than NCISA and TSA (mean differences = 0.75, 1.17; p = 0.049, 0.002, respectively). Additionally, regarding health status, NCISA had higher scores than TSA (mean differences = 0.94, p = 0.006).

4. Discussion

This survey reports some data from online research among Iranian individual and team sport athletes during the COVID-19 pandemic. A total of 1353 athletes from individual and team sports participated in this study. Changes in exercise before and during the COVID-19 pandemic showed that the intensity and frequency of exercise were higher before the COVID-19 pandemic than during it among all groups, apart from the intensity metric of TSA. Interestingly, intensity of TSA was higher during the COVID-19 pandemic but was not significant. These results are in line with most studies among the general population [5,26–28]. The scientific community has highlighted the real benefits of PA during the pandemic [29,30]; however, our results showed a reduction in exercise indexes among NCISA and CISA and exercise frequency among TSA. It seems that most team athletes may have performed home exercise, fitness, stretching, walking, and individual exercises at different intensities during this pandemic. Although the frequency of exercise decreased among them, in-depth checking of the present study results showed that the type of exercises had changed, which complied with exercise and PA recommendations during the coronavirus outbreak [31]. This experience could be due to essential changes in sports training schedules. Sports training was discontinued at the original coronavirus outbreak and research data were collected at that time; therefore, the present findings can be justified. This issue was consistent with Lim [32], who cited that many athletes attempt to maintain active lifestyles by themselves. Therefore, changes in daily life activities are necessary. It seems TSA may push themselves to keep fit and stay in shape by doing some other types of PA and exercise. It should also be noted that at the time of data collection of the present study, all places of sports activities, both individual and team, were closed, except for unorganized individual activities outdoors. However, at the same time, there were no nationwide closures for parks, shopping malls, etc., which may have affected the obtained results.

To address this issue, Mutz and Gerke [33] reported a significant decline in sport and exercise activities among Germans. Additionally, about one-third of the studied population reduced their sport and exercise activities, and only 6% intensified sport and exercise levels. They cited that this last group increased home-based workouts and outdoor endurance sports, while others did not adapt their sporting routines to the present conditions.

Based on Figure 1, all the positive moods were less than the negative ones among all groups. However, our results showed that CISA were more discouraged and vigorous. It seems that the type of sport could affect negative and positive mood states; sports in which the participants necessarily come into bodily contact with one another seemed to be more affected. Results of negative moods are consistent with recent research which indicates that the increasing menace of the epidemic has resulted in depression due to disrupted travel plans, social isolation, and media information overload [34].

In addition, positive relationships of exercise dependency with positive mood states and negative relationships with negative mood states were in line with a previous study [16]. They showed small to moderate correlations between exercise dependence with mood states. Previous research suggested that mood states could play a critical role in the development or the maintenance of exercise dependency [16,35,36]. The "affect regulation" hypothesis could justify this issue [36]. Therefore, PA results in improvements in positive mood states and decreases in negative mood states. As the exercise cycle continues, increased amounts of exercise are needed to experience improvement in affect and mood. On the other hand, lack of exercise can lead to a weakening of positive moods and an increase in negative moods.

In addition, exercise indexes were predicted by age, gender, adherence to quarantine, and exercise dependency in the three groups. Adherence to quarantine and exercise dependency were the best predictors of exercise frequency and intensity. Additionally, age and gender were able to predict the frequency and intensity of exercise in the CISA group.

It was further shown that CISA had unpleasant feelings of leaving exercise, and TSA had an unhealthier status than NCISA. Therefore, it seems that the nature of how an athlete interacts with other athletes may be important in the context of athletes' feelings during the COVID-19 pandemic.

Despite the new findings, several limitations warn against overgeneralization of the results. Firstly, the cross-sectional design of the study precludes conclusions about the studied variables. Secondly, although we used open- and closed-ended questions in this study, data collection through self-reporting may be biased. Thirdly, the present study data were collected only a few months after the onset of the COVID-19 pandemic; however, longitudinal studies seem to better clarify the changing trends of exercise indexes.

5. Conclusions

Among a large sample of Iranian athletes of different ages, gender, and sports, changing exercise indexes were not similar among groups; there was a dominant reduction pattern among all sports, and a non-significant increasing trend was also observed in team sports. Unlike previous studies, the present project did not focus only on the overall scores of negative or positive mood; it also presented new findings related to negative and positive mood subscales. Additionally, in this study, we showed that exercise dependency has a significant relationship with both positive and negative mood states. Finally, it was shown that with increasing exercise dependency, exercise intensity and frequency increased. Additionally, adherence to quarantine and exercise dependency were the best predictors of exercise indexes during the COVID-19 pandemic.

Author Contributions: Conceptualization, A.A. and H.R.; methodology, M.N.; software, Z.F.; S.H.Z.S. and E.K.; validation, A.A. and H.R.; formal analysis, S.H.Z.S.; investigation, Z.F.; resources, Z.F. and E.K.; data curation, S.H.Z.S.; writing—original draft preparation, Z.F.; writing—review and editing, A.A., G.B., H.R. and S.H.Z.S.; visualization, A.A. and G.B.; supervision, A.A.; project administration, A.A. and H.R. All authors have read and agreed to the published version of the manuscript.

Funding: This research received no external funding.

Institutional Review Board Statement: The Human Research Ethics Board at the Sport Sciences Research Institute of Iran approved the study (approval ID: IR.SSRC.REC.1399.070), which was performed in accordance with the seventh and current revision of the Declaration of Helsinki.

Informed Consent Statement: Informed consent was obtained from all subjects involved in the study. Individual and team sports athletes were approached via social network sites (SNS) to participate in the present online survey on past and current exercise patterns, mood states and exercise dependency. On the first page of the online survey, participants were informed about the aims of the study, the anonymous data gathering, the confidential data handling, and the ethical approval of the study. Next, to provide informed consent, participants clicked a box of agreement.

Data Availability Statement: The data presented in this study are available on request from the corresponding author.

Acknowledgments: We thank the Sport Sciences Research Institute of Iran for supporting this project. Additionally, the authors are grateful to all athletes who took part in the present study.

Conflicts of Interest: The authors declare no conflict of interest.

References

1. Pieh, C.; Budimir, S.; Probst, T. The effect of age, gender, income, work, and physical activity on mental health during coronavirus disease (COVID-19) lockdown in Austria. *J. Psychosom. Res.* **2020**, *136*, 110186. [CrossRef]
2. Qiu, J.; Shen, B.; Zhao, M.; Wang, Z.; Xie, B.; Xu, Y. A nationwide survey of psychological distress among Chinese people in the COVID-19 epidemic: Implications and policy recommendations. *Gen. Psychiatry* **2020**, *33*, e100213. [CrossRef] [PubMed]

3. Mehrsafar, A.H.; Gazerani, P.; Zadeh, A.M.; Sánchez, J.C.J. Addressing potential impact of COVID-19 pandemic on physical and mental health of elite athletes. *Brain Behav. Immun.* **2020**, *87*, 147–148. [CrossRef] [PubMed]
4. Jiao, W.Y.; Wang, L.N.; Liu, J.; Fang, S.F.; Jiao, F.Y.; Pettoello-Mantovani, M.; Somekh, E. Behavioral and emotional disorders in children during the COVID-19 epidemic. *J. Pediatr.* **2020**, *221*, 264–266. [CrossRef] [PubMed]
5. Ammar, A.; Brach, M.; Trabelsi, K.; Chtourou, H.; Boukhris, O.; Masmoudi, L.; Bouaziz, B.; Bentlage, E.; How, D.; Ahmed, M.; et al. Effects of COVID-19 Home Confinement on Eating Behavior and Physical Activity: Results of the ECLB-COVID19 International Online Survey. *Nutrients* **2020**, *12*, 1583. [CrossRef] [PubMed]
6. Iancheva, T.; Rogaleva, L.; GarcíaMas, A.; Olmedilla, A. Perfectionism, mood states, and coping strategies of sports students from Bulgaria and Russia during the pandemic COVID-19. *J. Appl. Sports Sci.* **2020**, *1*, 22–38. [CrossRef]
7. Jonker, L.; Elferink-Gemser, M.T.; Visscher, C. Differences in self-regulatory skills among talented athletes: The significance of competitive level and type of sport. *J. Sport Sci.* **2010**, *28*, 901–908. [CrossRef] [PubMed]
8. Nicholls, A.R.; Polman, R.; Levy, A.R.; Taylor, J.; Cobley, S. Stressors, coping, and coping effectiveness: Gender, type of sport, and skill differences. *J. Sport Sci.* **2007**, *25*, 1521–1530. [CrossRef]
9. Pluhar, E.; McCracken, C.; Griffith, K.L.; Christino, M.A.; Sugimoto, D.; Meehan, W.P., III. Team sport athletes may be less likely to suffer anxiety or depression than individual sport athletes. *J. Sports Sci. Med.* **2019**, *18*, 490.
10. Correia, M.; Rosado, A. Anxiety in athletes: Gender and type of sport differences. *Int. J. Psychol. Res.* **2019**, *12*, 9–17. [CrossRef] [PubMed]
11. Eagleton, J.R.; McKelvie, S.J.; De Man, A. Extraversion and neuroticism in team sport participants, individual sport participants, and nonparticipants. *Percept. Mot. Ski.* **2007**, *105*, 265–275. [CrossRef]
12. Ahmetov, I.I.; Borisov, O.V.; Semenova, E.A.; Andryushchenko, O.N.; Andryushchenko, L.B.; Generozov, E.V.; Pickering, C. Team sport, power, and combat athletes are at high genetic risk for coronavirus disease-2019 severity. *J. Sport Health Sci.* **2020**, *9*, 430. [CrossRef] [PubMed]
13. Köteles, F.; Kollsete, M.; Kollsete, H. Psychological concomitants of CrossFit training: Does more exercise really make your everyday psychological functioning better? *Kinesiol. Int. J. Fundam. Appl. Kinesiol.* **2016**, *48*, 39–48. [CrossRef]
14. Monteiro-Junior, R.S.; Rodrigues, V.D.; Campos, C.; Paes, F.; Murillo-Rodriguez, E.; Maranhão-Neto, G.A.; Machado, S. The role of physical activity on mood state and functional skills of elderly women. *Clin. Pract. Epidemiol. Ment. Health* **2017**, *13*, 125. [CrossRef] [PubMed]
15. Chan, J.S.; Liu, G.; Liang, D.; Deng, K.; Wu, J.; Yan, J.H. Special issue–therapeutic benefits of physical activity for mood: A systematic review on the effects of exercise intensity, duration, and modality. *J. Psychol.* **2019**, *153*, 102–125. [CrossRef]
16. Costa, S.; Hausenblas, H.A.; Oliva, P.; Cuzzocrea, F.; Larcan, R. The role of age, gender, mood states and exercise frequency on exercise dependence. *J. Behav. Addict.* **2013**, *2*, 216–223. [CrossRef] [PubMed]
17. Wang, C.; Pan, R.; Wan, X.; Tan, Y.; Xu, L.; Ho, C.S.; Ho, R.C. Immediate Psychological Responses and Associated Factors during the Initial Stage of the 2019 Coronavirus Disease (COVID-19) Epidemic among the General Population in China. *Int. J. Environ. Res. Public Health* **2020**, *17*, 1729. [CrossRef]
18. Wang, C.; Pan, R.; Wan, X.; Tan, Y.; Xu, L.; McIntyre, R.S.; Choo, F.N.; Tran, B.; Ho, R.; Sharma, V.K.; et al. A longitudinal study on the mental health of general population during the COVID-19 epidemic in China. *Brain Behav. Immun.* **2020**, *87*, 40–48. [CrossRef] [PubMed]
19. World Medical Association. World Medical Association Declaration of Helsinki: Ethical principles for medical research involving human subjects. *JAMA* **2013**, *310*, 2191–2194. [CrossRef] [PubMed]
20. Cho, M.H. Are Korean adults meeting the recommendations for physical activity during their leisure time? *J. Phys. Ther. Sci.* **2014**, *26*, 841–844. [CrossRef]
21. Cho, M.H. Preliminary reliability of the five items physical activity questionnaire. *J. Phys. Ther. Sci.* **2016**, *28*, 3393–3397. [CrossRef] [PubMed]
22. Terry, P.C.; Lane, A.M.; Fogarty, G.J. Construct validity of the Profile of Mood States-Adolescents for use with adults. *Psychol. Sport Exerc.* **2003**, *4*, 125–139. [CrossRef]
23. Petrowski, K.; Schmalbach, B.; Albani, C.; Beutel, M.E.; Brähler, E.; Zenger, M. Revised short screening version of the Profile of Mood States (POMS) from the German general population. *Manuscr. PLoS ONE* **2020**, *15*, e0234228.
24. Lin, S.; Hsiao, Y.Y.; Wang, M. Test review: The profile of mood states 2nd edition. *J. Psychoeduc. Assess.* **2014**, *32*, 273–277. [CrossRef]
25. Hauck, C.; Schipfer, M.; Ellrott, T.; Cook, B. "Always do your best!"—The relationship between food addiction, exercise dependence, and perfectionism in amateur athletes. *Ger. J. Exerc. Sport Res.* **2020**, *50*, 114–122. [CrossRef]
26. Sekulic, D.; Blazevic, M.; Gilic, B.; Kvesic, I.; Zenic, N. Prospective Analysis of Levels and Correlates of Physical Activity during COVID-19 Pandemic and Imposed Rules of Social Distancing; Gender Specific Study among Adolescents from Southern Croatia. *Sustainability* **2020**, *12*, 4072. [CrossRef]
27. Schuch, F.B.; Bulzing, R.A.; Meyer, J.; Vancampfort, D.; Firth, J.; Stubbs, B.; Grabovac, I.; Willeit, P.; Tavares, V.D.O.; Calegaro, V.C.; et al. Associations of moderate to vigorous physical activity and sedentary behavior with depressive and anxiety symptoms in self-isolating people during the COVID-19 pandemic: A cross-sectional survey in Brazil. *Psychiatry Res.* **2020**, *292*, 113339. [CrossRef]

28. Lesser, I.A.; Nienhuis, C.P. The Impact of COVID-19 on Physical Activity Behavior and Well-Being of Canadians. *Int. J. Environ. Res. Public Health* **2020**, *17*, 3899. [CrossRef] [PubMed]
29. Ricci, F.; Izzicupo, P.; Moscucci, F.; Sciomer, S.; Maffei, S.; Di Baldassarre, A.; Mattioli, A.V.; Gallina, S. Recommendations for Physical Inactivity and Sedentary Behavior During the Coronavirus Disease (COVID-19) Pandemic. *Front. Public Health* **2020**, *8*, 199. [CrossRef]
30. Yousfi, N.; Bragazzi, N.L.; Briki, W.; Zmijewski, P.; Chamari, K. The COVID-19 pandemic: How to maintain a healthy immune system during the lockdown–a multidisciplinary approach with special focus on athletes. *Biol. Sport* **2020**, *37*, 211. [CrossRef]
31. Zhu, W. Should, and how can, exercise be done during a coronavirus outbreak? An interview with Dr. Jeffrey, A. Woods. *J. Sport Health Sci.* **2020**, *9*, 105–107. [CrossRef]
32. Lim, M.A. Exercise addiction and COVID-19-associated restrictions. *J. Ment. Health* **2020**, *5*, 1–3. [CrossRef] [PubMed]
33. Mutz, M.; Gerke, M. Sport and exercise in times of self-quarantine: How Germans changed their behavior at the beginning of the Covid-19 pandemic. *Int. Rev. Sport Soc.* **2021**, *56*, 305–316. [CrossRef]
34. Ho, C.S.; Chee, C.Y.; Ho, R.C. Mental Health Strategies to Combat the Psychological Impact of COVID-19 beyond Paranoia and Panic. *Ann. Acad. Med.* **2020**, *49*, 155–160.
35. Berczik, K.; Szabó, A.; Griffiths, M.D.; Kurimay, T.; Kun, B.; Urbán, R.; Demetrovics, Z. Exercise addiction: Symptoms, diagnosis, epidemiology, and etiology. *Subst. Use Misuse* **2012**, *47*, 403–417. [CrossRef]
36. Hamer, M.; Karageorghis, C.I. Psychobiological mechanisms of exercise dependence. *Sports Med.* **2007**, *37*, 477–484. [CrossRef]

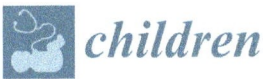

Article

Somatotype, Accumulated Workload, and Fitness Parameters in Elite Youth Players: Associations with Playing Position

Hadi Nobari [1,2,3,4,*], Rafael Oliveira [5,6,7], Filipe Manuel Clemente [8,9], Jorge Pérez-Gómez [2], Elena Pardos-Mainer [10] and Luca Paolo Ardigò [11]

1. Department of Physical Education and Sports, University of Granada, 18010 Granada, Spain
2. HEME Research Group, Faculty of Sport Sciences, University of Extremadura, 10003 Cáceres, Spain; jorgepg100@gmail.com
3. Sports Scientist, Sepahan Football Club, Isfahan 81887-78473, Iran
4. Department of Exercise Physiology, Faculty of Sport Sciences, University of Isfahan, Isfahan 81746-7344, Iran
5. Sports Science School of Rio Maior—Polytechnic Institute of Santarém, Av. Dr. Mário Soares, 2040-413 Rio Maior, Portugal; rafaeloliveira@esdrm.ipsantarem.pt
6. Research Centre in Sport Sciences, Health Sciences and Human Development, Quinta de Prados, Edifício Ciências de Desporto, 5001-801 Vila Real, Portugal
7. Life Quality Research Centre, Av. Dr. Mário Soares, 2040-413 Rio Maior, Portugal
8. Escola Superior Desporto e Lazer, Instituto Politécnico de Viana do Castelo, Rua Escola Industrial e Comercial de Nun'Álvares, 4900-347 Viana do Castelo, Portugal; Filipe.clemente5@gmail.com
9. Instituto de Telecomunicações, Delegação da Covilhã, 1049-001 Lisboa, Portugal
10. Health Sciences Faculty, Universidad San Jorge, Autov A23 km 299, 50830 Villanueva de Gállego, Spain; epardos@usj.es
11. Department of Neurosciences, Biomedicine and Movement Sciences, School of Exercise and Sport Science, University of Verona, 37131 Verona, Italy; luca.ardigo@univr.it
* Correspondence: hadi.nobari1@gmail.com

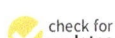

Citation: Nobari, H.; Oliveira, R.; Clemente, F.M.; Pérez-Gómez, J.; Pardos-Mainer, E.; Ardigò, L.P. Somatotype, Accumulated Workload, and Fitness Parameters in Elite Youth Players: Associations with Playing Position. *Children* **2021**, *8*, 375. https://doi.org/10.3390/children8050375

Academic Editor: Zoe Knowles

Received: 20 March 2021
Accepted: 6 May 2021
Published: 10 May 2021

Publisher's Note: MDPI stays neutral with regard to jurisdictional claims in published maps and institutional affiliations.

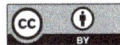

Copyright: © 2021 by the authors. Licensee MDPI, Basel, Switzerland. This article is an open access article distributed under the terms and conditions of the Creative Commons Attribution (CC BY) license (https://creativecommons.org/licenses/by/4.0/).

Abstract: The purpose of this study was three-fold: (1) to describe anthropometric, maturation, and somatotype differences of players based on playing positions; (2) to analyze variations of accumulated load training (AcL) and fitness parameters between playing positions; and finally (3) to explain the variation of maximal oxygen uptake (VO_{2max}) and peak power (PP) through the AcL, body fat (BF), maturity, somatotype and fitness levels. Twenty-seven male youth soccer players under-16 were divided by the following positions participated in this study: six central midfielders, four wingers (WG), five forwards, eight defenders, and four goalkeepers (GK). They were evaluated on two occasions: pre-season and after-season. Height, sitting height, body mass, BF, girths, percentage of BF (BF%), lean body mass, maturity, somatotype, sprint test, change of direction test, Yo-Yo intermittent recovery test level 1, Wingate, PP, VO_{2max} and fatigue index were assessed. Then, AcL was monitored during training sessions. The main results revealed significant differences between player positions for maturity offset ($p = 0.001$), for BF ($p = 0.006$), BF% ($p = 0.015$), and lean body mass kg ($p = 0.003$). Also, there were significant differences for AcL and fatigue index in pre-season between player positions ($p < 0.05$). In addition, there were some significant differences in pre- and after-season for VO_{2max} and PP between player positions ($p < 0.05$). In conclusion, GK showed higher values in anthropometric, body composition variables and maturity offset compared to the other positions, while WG presented lower levels of BF. In pre-season, there were more differences by player positions for the different variables analyzed than after-season that reinforces the tactical role of the positions, and the emphasis in increased load in the beginning of the season. This study could be used by coaches, staff, and researchers as a reference for athletes of the same sex, age, and competitive level.

Keywords: VO_{2max}; anthropometric; body composition; maturation; peak power; training load

1. Introduction

Soccer has specific requirements in different competitive levels, playing positions and age categories [1]. Soccer is multifactorial and conditioned by multiple variables such as anthropometric, body composition, somatotype, physical, physiological, and soccer-specific skills [2,3]. In this sense, scientific research regarding these topics has been developed, but still provides inclusive information [4]. With special regard to young age categories, there is a need to identify the differences between young soccer players, as any category can include different chronological and biological ages [5]. Therefore, anthropometry, somatotype and some fitness parameters are necessary to know the actual state of the player.

The identification of the somatotype helps to individualize exercise training programs which can differ by positions. Furthermore, this identification facilitates an understanding of the differences in adiposity level, robustness and musculoskeletal linearity [6]. Along with somatotype, anthropometric, body composition and physiologic variables are considered main areas regarding athletes' performance [7]. Chamari et al. [8] reinforce the finding that technical and tactical developments are influenced by morphological characteristics. In addition, the positions of youth soccer players can differ from others on body composition [9].

Soccer can be characterized by a predominant low-to-moderate intensity activity, interspaced with periods of high-intensity actions [10]. Therefore, soccer players depend on well-developed aerobic and anaerobic metabolisms to sustain the different efforts exerted in a match. Despite a predominance of aerobic activity, the most decisive skills, such as to perform a high jump, sprint or score a goal, come from the anaerobic system [11]. Therefore, soccer players need to develop different physical qualities to ensure the best performance during a match.

One of those qualities is the maximum rate of oxygen consumption (VO_{2max}). This is the physiological index most widely used for measuring aerobic fitness of soccer players and can be determined in both, laboratory and field tests. It helps to clarify the level of physical fitness and if it is high, it probably prevents or reduces the risk of injury [12–14].

A soccer game is composed of two parts of 45 min, where the movements, when playing on the field, are very complex and varied, so players require cruising capabilities throughout the game. For this reason, to achieve excellent physical fitness, a soccer player should have a high aerobic capacity [13,15].

In addition, coaches and sport science staff usually perform internal training load quantification to avoid high levels of fatigue and to reduce high risk of illness or injury [16,17]. Also, it allows a better individual and group training periodization [18,19]. Through the rating of perceived exertion (RPE) scale, it is possible to collect considerations regarding physiological characteristics applied during training sessions [20,21].

Furthermore, the knowledge of the aforementioned variables through the season is crucial and can impact training and performance during competition. Therefore, it is important to monitor, access and compare all variables during the different phases of the season. Thus, the literature is somewhat inconclusive about establishing differences in training load, anthropometric, body composition, somatotype, physical, physiological, and soccer-specific skills for player positions in youth players. Moreover, the majority of the studies split the different variables mentioned and do not use them simultaneously.

Therefore, the aims of this study were: (i) to describe baseline anthropometric, maturation, somatotype and fitness parameters differences of players based on playing positions; (ii) to analyze variations of accumulated load training (AcL) between playing positions for periods analyzed; and finally (iii) to explain the variation of VO_{2max} and peak power (PP) through the AcL, body fat (BF), maturity, somatotype, and baseline fitness levels.

2. Materials and Methods
2.1. The Experimental Approach to the Problem

The present study consists of two parts: the first is a semi-experimental design with pre- and post-test; the second is a cohort with daily monitoring for 18 weeks in the competitive season. They practiced 5 sessions a week with one match. The team usually performed one resistance training session, one short-speed training session, agility, and small-sided games (SSG) with skill and tactical training per week. The season was divided into two equal periods of eight weeks: early-season and end-season. The first assessment was in the week before starting the league (pre-season), and the second measurement was done after the league (post-season). Players were assessed on four consecutive days. Anthropometric and body composition were assessed in one day (e.g., height, sitting height, body mass, BF, and girths) then based on this information the percentage of body fat (BF%), lean body mass (LBM), the maturity and somatotype of the players were calculated. The next day, the sprint and change of direction (COD) tests were performed. In the following day, Wingate test was performed to obtain PP and fatigue index (FI), which was considered as a criterion for assessing the anaerobic capacity of players, and on the last day, the Yo-Yo intermittent recovery test level 1 (YYIRT1) was performed to estimate the aerobic power of the players along with the calculation of the VO_{2max}. All tests were performed for each participant under similar environmental conditions and in the same order. Thirty minutes after each training session, all players reported load of training, then each 'training load' was used with training time for calculating AcL for the two periods.

2.2. Participants

Twenty-seven elite soccer players, belonging to the same national under-16 team competing in the national league, were evaluated for 18 weeks during a competitive season. In total, 76 training sessions and 16 competitive matches were held. To analyze the differences between player positions, they were organized by six central midfielders (CM) with maturity offset 1.72 ± 0.18 years (yrs), four wingers (WG) with maturity offset 1.55 ± 0.17 yrs, five forwards (FW) with maturity offset 2.08 ± 0.33 yrs, eight defenders (DF) with maturity offset 1.94 ± 0.19 yrs, and four goalkeepers (GK) with maturity offset 2.38 ± 0.32 yrs. Inclusion and exclusion criteria in this study were: (i) players who participated in at least 90% of training seasons; (ii) players that did not participate in another training plan along with this study; (iii) each player who was not participating in the match during a week was practicing a separate session, without the ball or through SSG. Before starting this study, explanations about the different phases of the research were given to all participants along with their parents. Also, they were informed of the potential risks and benefits of participating in the study. The study was conducted in accordance with the Declaration of Helsinki; players and their parents given and signed their informed consent to participate in this study, which was approved by the Ethics Committee of the Sport Sciences Research Institute (IR.SSRC.REC.1399.060).

We calculated an a-posteriori estimation of sample size, accepting an alpha risk of 0.05 and a beta risk of 0.2 in a two-sided test; 4 players are necessary for each group to be recognized as statistically significant, with a minimum difference of 10.06 units between any pair of groups, assuming that 5 groups exist. The common deviation is assumed to be 3.64. A drop-out rate of 0% was anticipated.

2.3. Procedures

2.3.1. Anthropometric and Body Composition

To measure the standing height, participants stood in the stadiometer without shoes and socks. They kept heels, hips, shoulder blades and back of the head as close as possible to the stadiometer, and then feet were placed beside each other. For sitting height, participants sat on a 50 cm bench and brought their buttocks as close as possible to the stadiometer, holding their upper body straight and placing their hands on their feet, then their heights were assessed. The distance between the highest point of the head and the bench, which was at 50 cm, was calculated as sitting height. For this measurement, portable stadiometer SECA (Model 213, Germany) was used with an accuracy of 5 mm.

For measuring maturity offset and age at peak high velocity (PHV), we used the formula: Maturity offset = $-9.236 + 0.0002708$ (leg length $\times$ sitting height) $- 0.001663$ (age $\times$ leg length) $+ 0.007216$ (age $\times$ sitting height) $+ 0.02292$ (Weight by Height ratio), R = 0.94, R2 = 0.891, and SEE = 0.592) and for leg length = Standing Height (cm) $-$ Sitting height (cm) [22]. To measure weight, participants only wore one pair of sports shorts for body weight on the scale SECA (model 813, England), with an accuracy of ± 0.1 kg.

The subcutaneous fat thickness of the seven points of the body including the chest, abdomen, thigh, triceps, subscapular, suprailiac and midaxillary were calculated for body density (BD) by Jackson and Pollock method and for BD and BF% with Brozek's formula [23]. Skin thickness was obtained by calibrating Lafayette Instrument Company (Lafayette, IN, USA) with an accuracy of 0.1 mm. All measurements were performed twice on the right side of the body, the final score recorded with the mean of two measurements. The technical standard error of subcutaneous fat measurement was performed according to previous studies [24]. Other anthropometric measurements such as girths (cm), relaxed arm, flexed arm, chest, waist, hip, upper thigh, mid-thigh, calf and abdomen were measured using the techniques provided by the International Society for the Advancement of Kinanthropometry Advance also used in previous study [25]. The technical error of measurement, inter- and intra-observer, was lower than 3% for the other variables.

2.3.2. Somatotype

Body somatotype, the three-dimensional distance from a profile to the mean of all profiles (endomorph, mesomorph and ectomorph) and height to weight ratio (HWR), according to Carter and Heath [5], were calculated from anthropometric measures including height, weight, four skinfold thickness (triceps, subscapular, supraspinal, and medial calf), two epicondylar breadths (humerus and femur) and two girths (upper arm flexed and tensed, and calf). The somatotypes were plotted in agreement with previous studies [25,26] on a two-dimensional grid system somatochart using the appropriate software https://www.somatotype.org/ (accessed on 20 March 2021) (Somatotype 1.2 software). All measurements were performed by an expert with five years of background in this area. All anthropometric measurements were performed in the morning [25].

2.3.3. Change of Direction Test

Players did the "modified 505 agility test" [27]. A photo-finish system recorded the time of a complete 5 m turn (2 × 5 m). All procedures were described in our previous study [28]. The best of the efforts performed was used for statistical analysis. The intra-class correlation coefficient (ICC) in this study was equal to two replicates of 0.90 in this test.

2.3.4. Sprint Test

For sprint test a digital timer connected to two photocells was placed at hip height, and after 10-min specific warm-up subjects stood 70 cm before the start line. To calculate the sprint time [29], the test was performed at a distance of 30 m. The best value obtained from 3 trials was used for statistical analysis. Subjects had to rest for at least 3 min between each trial. All phases of testing were monitored by the coach. In this study, COD and sprint tests were performed with the Newtest Powertimer 300-series testing system (Tyrnävä, Finland). The ICC in this study was equal to two replicates of 0.87 in this test.

2.3.5. Anaerobic Power

The Wingate test [30,31] was selected to measure anaerobic power (PP and FI). After giving a warm-up to subjects, the seat height was adjusted so that knee flexion degrees were 170–175, with leg extended fully. At first, to determine the repetition per minute (RPM), the subject began to pedal at their maximum speed for 5 s. RPM was recorded immediately from the ergometer monitor. According to the calculated value and body mass (75 g per kg of body mass), the resistance load of the test was set. The testing procedure consisted of the participants performing a 10-s countdown phase and a 30-s quick pedaling phase; all subjects were verbally encouraged to continue to pedal as fast as they could for the entire 30 s. Ultimately, the desired indicators were calculated using the Wingate power software program of the Monark model 894-E ergometer (Vansbro, Sweden). The ICC in this study was equal to two replicates of 0.94 in this test.

2.3.6. Aerobic Power Test

To evaluate the aerobic power, the YYIRT1 was used and then, VO_{2max} was calculated based on the following formula: VO_{2max} (mL·kg^{-1}·min^{-1}) = YYIRT1 distance (m) × 0.0084 + 36.4 [32]. The ICC in this study was equal to two replicates of 0.86 in this test.

2.3.7. Monitoring Accumulated Training Load

Players were monitored daily for their RPE using the CR-10 Borg's scale, a valid and reliable scale to estimate the intensity of a session [33]. To the question "How intense was your session?" players answered in the interval of number zero for the day without training, 1 for minimum effort and 10 for maximal effort. Players provided responses 30 min after the end of the training session [12,34]. Additionally, the duration of the training sessions (in minutes) was recorded for each player. As a measure of internal load, the s-RPE was calculated by multiplying the score in the CR-10 scale by the duration of the session in minutes [35,36]. Players were previously familiarized with the scale through spending two years at the club. In this study, the AcL (for training and competition) was used for 18 weeks. These weeks of the full competitive season were divided into two periods: early-season, from week (W) 1 to W8 (includes 8 competitions and 39 practice sessions); and end-season, from W9 to W16 (includes 8 competitions and 37 practice sessions).

2.3.8. Statistical Analysis

Statistical analyses were performed using SPSS (version 23.0, IBM SPSS Inc., Chicago, IL, USA) and Graph-Pad Prism 8.0.1 (GraphPad Software Inc, San Diego, California, CA, USA). The significance level was set at $p < 0.05$. Data are presented as mean and standard deviation (SD). Then, inferential tests were executed. Changes between the two in-season periods were assessed using a repeated-measures analysis of variance (ANOVA), followed by Bonferroni post hoc test for pairwise comparisons. Partial eta squared (ηp^2) was calculated as effect size of the repeated-measures ANOVA. Besides this, a one-way ANOVA was applied to compare the different assessment variables, by playing position, in each season period. Hedge's g effect sizes with 95% confidence interval were also calculated to determine the magnitude of pairwise comparisons for between-period comparisons. The Hopkins' thresholds for effect size statistics were used, as follows: ≤0.2, trivial; >0.2, small; >0.6, moderate; >1.2, large; >2.0, very large; and >4.0, nearly perfect [37]. Then, multiple linear regression analysis between the percentage of change in fitness levels include VO_{2max} and PP which were calculated by this formula ([POST − PRE]/PRE TEST) × 100). The independent variables considered for multiple linear regression were AcL, BF%, maturity, somatotype, and baseline fitness levels in the soccer players. The Akaike information criterion (AIC) for each model's regression was calculated. Multiple linear regression analysis and AIC were calculated with the R software version 4.0.2 (22 June 2020; R Foundation for Statistical Computing, Vienna, Austria). The test-retest reliability assessments, ICCs, were used. The ICC >0.7 was suitable [38]. G-Power software (University of Düsseldorf, Düsseldorf, Germany) was used for the sample size calculated with the design of the study.

3. Results

Table 1 shows comparisons between the different playing positions for anthropometric, maturity, body composition and somatotype variables. The most important results of one-way ANOVA showed significant differences between playing positions for maturity offset ($p = 0.001$). Hence, goalkeeper (GK) presented a significantly greater value than central midfielders (CM) ($p = 0.007$; CI95% = 0.14–1.18) and wingers (WG) ($p = 0.002$; CI95% = 0.25–1.40). Also, defender (DF) presented a significantly greater value than WG ($p = 0.032$; CI95% = 0.03–1.02). For body composition variables, it shows significant differences in (body fat) BF kg ($p = 0.006$), BF% ($p = 0.015$), and lean body mass (LBM; $p = 0.003$). Those differences were found between playing positions for BF%, where WG presented a significantly smaller BF% than CM and GK, respectively ($p = 0.022$; CI95% = −11.02–−0.59

and $p = 0.025$; CI95% = -11.98–-0.55). For LBM, GK presented a significantly greater value than CM and WG ($p = 0.002$; CI95% = 3.94–22 and $p = 0.022$; CI95% = 1.09–20.87), respectively. Further results are shown in Table 1.

Table 1. Absolute size characteristic, body composition, somatotype and anthropometric of soccer player by playing positions.

Characteristic		Position										p
		CM (n = 6)		WG (n = 4)		DF (n = 8)		FW (n = 5)		GK (n = 4)		
		Mean	SD	Mean	SD	Mean	SD	Mean	SD	Mean	SD	
Anthropometric	Age (yrs)	15.38	0.25	15.30	0.36	15.48	0.19	15.54	0.21	15.48	0.36	0.627
	Height (cm)	170.50 *	2.07	170.50 *	2.89	173.80 *	5.12	174.00 *	4.07	181.75	2.75	0.001 €
	Weight (kg)	58.34 *	2.17	56.88 *	4.76	62.98 *	6.35	63.38 *	4.70	73.44	6.43	0.001 €
	Career (yrs)	7.00	1.26	5.25	1.26	6.20	1.79	6.00	1.51	7.25	1.71	0.308
Maturations (yrs)	PHV	13.67	0.22	13.75	0.40	13.54	0.29	13.48	0.41	13.05	0.58	0.115
	Maturity offset	1.72 *	0.18	1.55 *	0.17	1.94 #	0.19	2.08	0.33	2.38	0.32	0.001 €
Body compositions	BF%	10.86 #	2.37	5.06 *	1.00	8.73	0.63	8.71	3.56	11.32	2.95	0.015 €
	BF (kg)	6.31	1.26	2.85 *	0.43	5.52	0.88	5.54	2.33	8.43	2.86	0.006 €
	LBM (kg)	52.04 *	3.02	54.03 *	5.01	57.46	5.51	57.84	4.61	65.01	4.16	0.003 €
Somatotype	HWR	43.97	0.28	44.46	0.43	43.74	1.17	43.83	0.46	43.36	1.03	0.306
	Endomorph	3.77 #	0.52	2.05	0.49	3.06	0.36	3.03	0.96	3.33	0.83	0.020 €
	Mesomorph	2.10	0.89	2.33	0.13	2.64	0.89	3.00	1.03	2.78	0.52	0.360
	Ectomorph	3.62	0.23	3.90	0.47	3.44	0.86	3.44	0.37	3.18	0.76	0.428
Girths (cm)	Relaxed arm	23.00	2.02	22.43	0.79	23.72	1.29	24.35	2.18	25.88	1.18	0.068
	Flexed arm	24.83	2.27	24.78	0.67	26.14	1.28	26.40	2.78	27.70	1.06	0.201
	Chest	78.92	4.24	77.75	3.77	81.80	2.80	77.08	20.68	87.08	3.34	0.709
	Waist	72.12	4.95	69.58	3.58	72.78	3.47	72.53	6.45	79.18	3.92	0.119
	Hip	49.77	2.76	46.53 *	0.81	50.52	2.03	51.63	4.18	54.40	4.12	0.030 €
	Upper thigh	85.42	4.40	83.00 *	1.22	89.22	3.55	89.65	4.70	92.35	5.20	0.024 €
	Mid-thigh	45.93	1.46	43.60	1.19	46.34	3.57	48.86	4.16	48.60	4.76	0.129
	Calf	33.17	1.37	32.28	1.23	34.64	2.18	35.43	2.13	36.75	4.19	0.057
	Abdominal	68.78	3.49	67.88	2.02	70.72	2.04	70.88	8.26	72.75	6.95	0.736

CM, central midfielders; WG, winger; FW, forward; DF, Defender; GK, goalkeeper; PHV = Peak height velocity; BF = Body fat; LBM = lean body mass; HWR = Height to weight ratio; yrs, years; SD, standard deviation. € Represents a statistically significant difference between groups to one-way ANOVA ($p < 0.05$); * Represents a statistically significant difference compared with goalkeepers ($p < 0.05$); # Represents a statistically significant difference compared with wingers ($p < 0.05$).

Figure 1 shows the somatotype according to divided playing positions. The somatotype ($p = 0.020$) only showed significant differences between playing positions for endomorph where CM presented a significant greater ($p = 0.011$; CI95% = 0.29–3.15) than WG.

Significant differences between season periods in accumulated load training (AcL) demonstrated main effects of time ($F (1, 7.73) p = 0.011$; $\eta_p^2 = 0.261$) and group effect ($F (4, 3.43) p = 0.025$; $\eta_p^2 = 0.384$). Post hoc tests using the Bonferroni correction revealed a significant increase in AcL. There was an only a significant difference between early-season and end-season in forwards (FW) ($p = 0.043$; CI95% = 125.17–4942.44). Tables 2 and 3 show comparisons between the different playing positions for fitness status in pre- and post-season, respectively. This variable was also the analysis of one-way ANOVA with a comparison between different playing position groups in each test time, and it was demonstrated that there was a difference in AcL compared to early-season (WG vs. FW: $p < 0.021$, $g = 3.09$; WG vs. GK: $p < 0.001$, $g = 2.35$; and DF vs. GK: $p < 0.050$, $g = 1.32$). However, no differences were found between playing position in end-season period for AcL.

There was a significant main effect of time for VO$_{2max}$ ($F (1, 10.37) p = 0.004$; $\eta_p^2 = 0.320$) and group effect ($F (4, 9.45) p < 0.001$ $\eta_p^2 = 0.632$). Post hoc analysis revealed VO$_{2max}$ was significantly greater at post-season in CM ($p = 0.042$; CI95% = 0.08–3.18) and DF ($p = 0.048$; CI95% = 0.01–1.95). Also, between player positions, this variable demonstrated that there was a significant difference within the pre-season (CM vs. GK: $p \leq 0.001$, $g = 4.10$; WG vs. GK: $p \leq 0.001$, $g = 6.75$; FW vs. GK: $p < 0.002$, $g = 3.11$; and DF vs. GK: $p < 0.001$, $g = 2.57$) as well as in the post-season (CM vs. GK: $p \leq 0.001$, $g = 3.88$; WG vs. GK: $p < 0.003$, $g = 5.66$; FW vs. GK: $p < 0.003$, $g = 2.83$; and DF vs. GK: $p < 0.001$, $g = 2.57$).

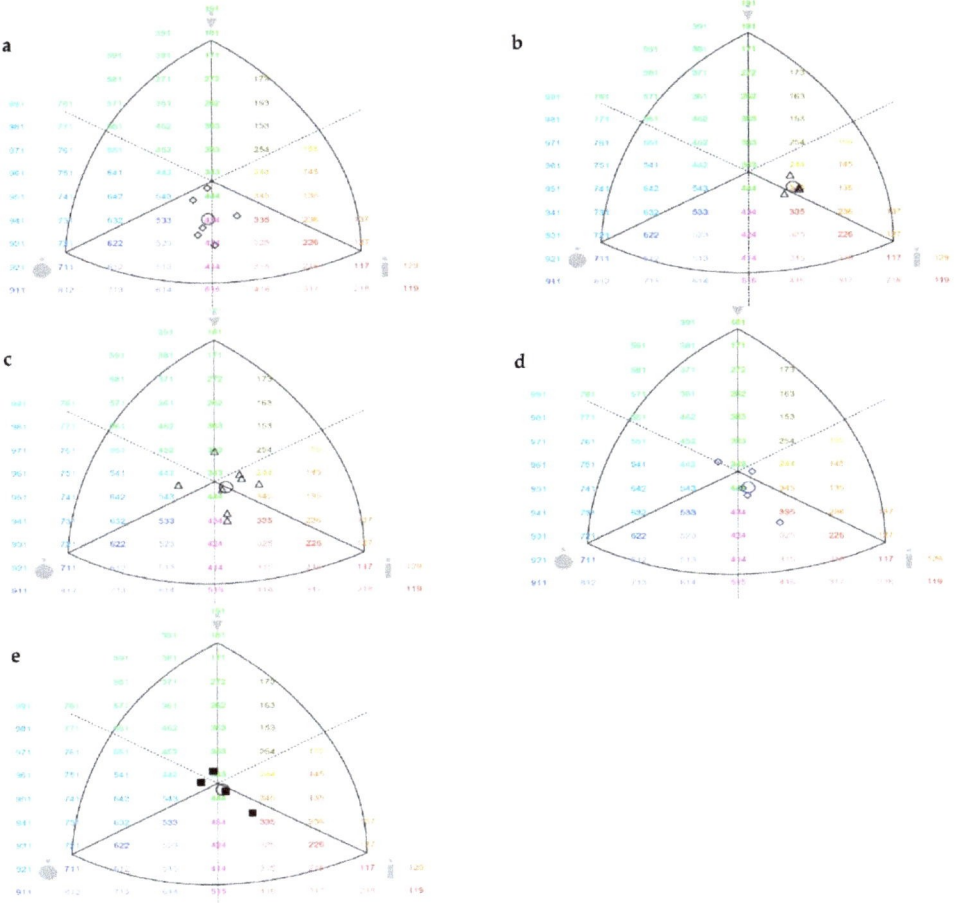

Figure 1. Individual somatotypes by the 2-D somatochart (**a**) Central midfielder, (**b**) Winger, (**c**) Defender, (**d**) Forward, (**e**) Goalkeeper. O = the mean somatotype.

Peak power (PP) levels demonstrated main effects of time (F (1, 22.21) $p \leq 0.001$; $\eta_p^2 = 0.502$) and group effect (F (4, 9.12) $p \leq 0.001$; $\eta_p^2 = 0.624$). Post hoc tests using the Bonferroni correction revealed a significant increase in PP between pre-season and post-season in CM ($p = 0.024$; CI95% = 19.93–183.40), DF ($p = 0.047$; CI95% = 1.11–132.39) and GK ($p = 0.041$; CI95% = 3.41–80.59). Also, between player positions, this variable demonstrated that there was a significant difference in the pre-season (WG vs. FW: $p = 0.001$, $g = 3.93$; FW vs. DF: $p = 0.009$, $g = -1.75$; and FW vs. GK: $p = 0.001$, $g = -4.81$) and ultimately, in the post-season (CM vs. FW: $p = 0.008$, $g = 1.83$; WG vs. FW: $p = 0.002$, $g = 2.91$; FW vs. DF: $p = 0.004$, $g = -1.93$; and FW vs. GK: $p = 0.001$, $g = -3.33$). Further results regarding FI are shown in Tables 2 and 3.

Table 2. Between-group comparisons for accumulated load and fitness parameters between playing positions in pre-season.

Variables	Groups		Mean SD	Collation	M Diff	95% CI for Diff	p	Hedge's g 95% CI
AcL (A.U.)	HB	M	10,182.0	HB vs. WG	−1828.5	[−4119.6 to 462.6]	0.209	−2.39 [−4.04 to −0.8]
		SD	549.7	HB vs. FW	832.4	[−1316.8 to 2981.6]	>0.999	1.25 [−0.04 to 2.6]
	WG	M	12,010.5	HB vs. DF	−275.1	[−2192.0 to 1641.7]	>0.999	−0.23 [−1.3 to 0.8]
		SD	873.6	HB vs. GK	1897.0	[−394.1 to 4188.1]	0.170	1.49 [0.1 to 2.9]
	FW	M	9349.6	WG vs. FW	2660.9 *	[280.0 to 5041.8]	0.021 #	3.09 [1.2 to 5.0]
		SD	671.3	WG vs. DF	1553.4	[−620.1 to 3726.9]	0.363	1.13 [−0.2 to 2.4]
	DF	M	10,457.1	WG vs. GK	3725.5 *	1215.8 to 6235.2]	0.001 #	2.35 [0.6 to 4.2]
		SD	1405.8	FW vs. DF	−1107.5	[−3130.9 to 915.9]	>0.999	−0.86 [−2.0 to 0.3]
	GK	M	8285.0	FW vs. GK	1064.6	[−1316.3 to 3445.5]	>0.999	0.76 [−0.6 to 2.1]
		SD	1737.4	DF vs. GK	2172.1	[−1.4 to 4345.6]	0.050 #	1.32 [0.01 to 2.6]
VO$_{2max}$ (mL·kg^{-1}·min^{-1})	HB	M	49.9	HB vs. WG	−0.2	[−5.1 to 4.7]	>0.999	−0.08 [−1.4 to 1.2]
		SD	2.3	HB vs. FW	1.3	[−3.3 to 5.8]	>0.999	0.46 [−0.7 to 1.7]
	WG	M	50.1	HB vs. DF	1.3	[−2.8 to 5.3]	>0.999	0.42 [−0.7 to 1.5]
		SD	1.5	HB vs. GK	8.5 *	[3.6 to 13.3]	<0.001 #	4.10 [1.9 to 6.3]
	FW	M	48.7	WG vs. FW	1.4	[−3.6 to 6.5]	>0.999	0.57 [−0.8 to 1.9]
		SD	2.7	WG vs. DF	1.5	[−3.2 to 6.1]	>0.999	0.50 [−0.7 to 1.7]
	DF	M	48.6	WG vs. GK	8.6 *	[3.3 to 14.0]	<0.001 #	6.75 [3.2 to 10.3]
		SD	3.1	FW vs. DF	0.0	[−4.3 to 4.3]	>0.999	0.01 [−1.1 to 1.1]
	GK	M	41.5	FW vs. GK	7.2 *	[2.1 to 12.3]	0.002 #	3.11 [1.2 to 5.1]
		SD	0.5	DF vs. GK	7.2 *	[2.6 to 11.8]	0.001 #	2.57 [0.9 to 4.2]
Sprint (m.s)	HB	M	3.44	HB vs. WG	−0.06	[−0.76 to 0.63]	>0.999	−0.17 [−1.4 to 1.1]
		SD	0.38	HB vs. FW	0.08	[−0.57 to 0.73]	>0.999	0.19 [−1.0 to 1.4]
	WG	M	3.51	HB vs. DF	0.03	[−0.55 to 0.61]	>0.999	0.07 [−0.9 to 1.1]
		SD	0.18	HB vs. GK	0.29	[−0.41 to 0.98]	>0.999	0.76 [−0.6 to 2.1]
	FW	M	3.36	WG vs. FW	0.14	[−0.58 to 0.86]	>0.999	0.39 [−0.9 to 1.7]
		SD	0.40	WG vs. DF	0.09	[−0.57 to 0.75]	>0.999	0.26 [−0.9 to 1.5]
	DF	M	3.42	WG vs. GK	0.35	[−0.41 to 1.11]	>0.999	1.33 [−0.2 to 2.9]
		SD	0.37	FW vs. DF	−0.05	[−0.67 to 0.56]	>0.999	−0.13 [−1.3 to 0.9]
	GK	M	3.16	FW vs. GK	0.20	[−0.52 to 0.93]	>0.999	0.52 [−0.8 to 1.9]
		SD	0.27	DF vs. GK	0.26	[−0.40 to 0.92]	>0.999	0.70 [−0.5 to 1.9]
COD (m.s)	HB	M	1.97	HB vs. WG	0.07	[−0.27 to 0.42]	>0.999	0.27 [−1.0 to 1.5]
		SD	0.22	HB vs. FW	0.13	[−0.19 to 0.46]	>0.999	0.67 [−0.6 to 1.9
	WG	M	1.90	HB vs. DF	0.06	[−0.23 to 0.35]	>0.999	0.35 [−0.7 to 1.4]
		SD	0.30	HB vs. GK	0.04	[−0.31 to 0.38]	>0.999	0.18 [−1.1 to 1.5]
	FW	M	1.83	WG vs. FW	0.06	[−0.30 to 0.42]	>0.999	0.25 [−1.1 to 1.6]
		SD	0.13	WG vs. DF	−0.01	[−0.34 to 0.31]	>0.999	−0.08 [−1.3 to 1.1]
	DF	M	1.91	WG vs. GK	−0.04	[−0.41 to 0.34]	>0.999	−0.15 [−1.5 to 1.2]
		SD	0.08	FW vs. DF	−0.08	[−0.38 to 0.23]	>0.999	−0.69 [−1.8 to 0.5]
	GK	M	1.93	FW vs. GK	−0.10	[−0.46 to 0.26]	>0.999	−0.75 [−2.1 to 0.6]
		SD	0.10	DF vs. GK	−0.02	[−0.35 to 0.30]	>0.999	−0.23 [−1.4 to 0.9]

Table 2. Cont.

Variables	Groups		Mean SD	Collation	M Diff	95% CI for Diff	p	Hedge's g 95% CI
Peak Power (w)	HB	M	699.8	HB vs. WG	−130.7	[−321.4 to 60.1]	0.440	−1.32 [−2.7 to 0.1]
		SD	104.9	HB vs. FW	168.2	[−10.7 to 347.2]	0.077	1.65 [0.3 to 3.0]
	WG	M	830.5	HB vs. DF	−38.7	[−198.2 to 120.9]	>0.999	−0.31 [−1.4 to 0.8]
		SD	53.7	HB vs. GK	−145.9	[−336.6 to 44.8]	0.261	−1.59 [−3.0 to −0.1]
	FW	M	531.6	WG vs. FW	298.9 *	[100.7 to 497.1]	0.001 #	3.93 [1.7 to 6.2]
		SD	76.4	WG vs. DF	92.0	[−88.9 to 272.9]	>0.999	0.78 [−0.5 to 2.0]
	DF	M	738.5	WG vs. GK	−15.3	[−224.2 to 193.7]	>0.999	−0.34 [−1.7 to 1.1]
		SD	125.5	FW vs. DF	−206.9	[−375.3 to −38.5]	0.009 #	−1.75 [−3.1 to −0.4]
	GK	M	845.8	FW vs. GK	−314.2	[−512.6 to −115.9]	0.001 #	−4.81 [−7.4 to −2.2]
		SD	8.7	DF vs. GK	−107.3	[−288.2 to 73.7]	0.780	−0.94 [−2.2 to 0.3]
Fatigue index (%)	HB	M	39.4	HB vs. WG	−2.8	[−6.5 to 0.8]	0.250	−1.39 [−2.8 to 0.01]
		SD	1.7	HB vs. FW	−0.5	[−3.9 to 3.0]	>0.999	−0.23 [−1.4 to 0.9]
	WG	M	42.3	HB vs. DF	−1.9	[−5.0 to 1.1]	0.595	−1.01 [−2.1 to 0.1]
		SD	2.0	HB vs. GK	−3.8	[−7.5 to −0.2]	0.036 #	−2.34 [−3.9 to −0.7]
	FW	M	39.9	WG vs. FW	2.4	[−1.5 to 6.2]	0.680	0.98 [−0.4 to 2.4]
		SD	2.2	WG vs. DF	0.9	[−2.6 to 4.4]	>0.999	0.42 [−0.8 to 1.6]
	DF	M	41.4	WG vs. GK	−1	[−5.0 to 3.0]	>0.999	−0.55 [−1.9 to 0.9]
		SD	1.9	FW vs. DF	−1.5	[−4.7 to 1.8]	>0.999	−0.69 [−1.8 to 0.5]
	GK	M	43.3	FW vs. GK	−3.4	[−7.2 to 0.5]	0.121	−1.68 [−3.2 to −0.2]
		SD	1.0	DF vs. GK	−1.9	[−5.4 to 1.6]	>0.999	−1.05 [−2.3 to 0.2]

M, Mean; diff, difference; AcL, accumulated load training; COD = change of direction; VO_{2max}, maximal oxygen consumption; CM, central midfielder; WG, winger; FW, forward; DF, Defender; GK, goalkeeper; SD, standard deviation; A.U., arbitrary units; CI, confidence interval, and p, p-value at alpha level 0.05; Hedge's g (95% CI), Hedge's g effect size magnitude with 95% confidence interval. * The mean difference is significant at the 0.05 levels; # Indicates a significant difference between the groups with Bonferroni at the 0.05 levels.

Table 3. Between-group comparisons for accumulated load and fitness parameters between playing positions in after-season.

Variables	Groups		Mean SD	Collation	M Diff	95% CI for Diff	p	Hedge's g 95% CI
AcL (A.U.)	HB	M	11800.2	HB vs. WG	105.9	[−3938.6 to 4150.4]	>0.999	0.05 [−1.2 to 1.3]
		SD	2087.2	HB vs. FW	−83.4	[−3877.5 to 3710.6]	>0.999	−0.04 [−1.2 to 1.2]
	WG	M	11694.3	HB vs. DF	872.3	[−2511.6 to 4256.2]	>0.999	0.45 [−0.6 to 1.5]
		SD	1307.2	HB vs. GK	3456.7	[−587.8 to 7501.2]	0.141	1.19 [−0.2 to 2.6]
	FW	M	11883.6	WG vs. FW	−189.4	[−4392.5 to 4013.8]	>0.999	−0.11 [−1.4 to 1.2]
		SD	1750.6	WG vs. DF	766.4	[−3070.6 to 4603.3]	>0.999	0.48 [−0.7 to 1.7]
	DF	M	10927.9	WG vs. GK	3350.8	[−1079.8 to 7781.3]	0.276	1.15 [−0.3 to 2.7]
		SD	1536.7	FW vs. DF	955.7	[−2616.3 to 4527.7]	>0.999	0.55 [−0.6 to 1.7]
	GK	M	8343.5	FW vs. GK	3540.1	[−663.1 to 7743.3]	0.154	1.24 [−0.2 to 2.7]
		SD	3321.4	DF vs. GK	2584.4	[−1252.6 to 6421.3]	0.474	1.07 [−0.2 to 2.3]
VO_{2max} (mL·kg^{-1}·min^{-1})	HB	M	51.6	HB vs. WG	1.4	[−4.0 to 6.8]	>0.999	0.55 [−0.7 to 1.8]
		SD	2.7	HB vs. FW	1.9	[−3.1 to 7.0]	>0.999	0.61 [−0.6 to 1.8]
	WG	M	50.1	HB vs. DF	1.9	[−2.6 to 6.4]	>0.999	0.59 [−0.5 to 1.7]
		SD	1.5	HB vs. GK	9.6 *	[4.2 to 15.0]	<0.001 #	3.88 [1.8 to 5.9]
	FW	M	49.6	WG vs. FW	0.5	[−5.1 to 6.1]	>0.999	0.18 [−1.1 to 1.5]
		SD	3.1	WG vs. DF	0.5	[−4.6 to 5.6]	>0.999	0.17 [−1.0 to 1.4]
	DF	M	49.6	WG vs. GK	8.2 *	[2.3 to 14.1]	0.003 #	5.66 [2.6 to 8.8]
		SD	3.2	FW vs. DF	0.0	[−4.7 to 4.8]	>0.999	0.00 [−1.1 to 1.1]
	GK	M	41.9	FW vs. GK	7.7 *	[2.1 to 13.3]	0.003 #	2.83 [0.9 to 4.7]
		SD	1.0	DF vs. GK	7.7 *	[2.6 to 12.8]	0.001 #	2.57 [0.9 to 4.2]

Table 3. Cont.

Variables	Groups		Mean SD	Collation	M Diff	95% CI for Diff	p	Hedge's g 95% CI
Sprint (m.s)	HB	M	3.36	HB vs. WG	−0.20	[−0.9 to 0.5]	>0.999	−0.47 [−1.8 to 0.8]
		SD	0.44	HB vs. FW	0.03	[−0.6 to 0.7]	>0.999	0.07 [−1.1 to 1.3]
	WG	M	3.55	HB vs. DF	−0.02	[−0.6 to 0.6]	>0.999	−0.05 [−1.1 to 1.0]
		SD	0.24	HB vs. GK	0.16	[−0.5 to 0.9]	>0.999	0.37 [−0.9 to 1.6]
	FW	M	3.32	WG vs. FW	0.23	[−0.5 to 1.0]	>0.999	0.62 [−0.7 to 1.9]
		SD	0.38	WG vs. DF	0.18	[−0.5 to 0.8]	>0.999	0.57 [−0.7 to 1.8]
	DF	M	3.38	WG vs. GK	0.36	[−0.4 to 1.1]	>0.999	1.19 [−0.3 to 2.7]
		SD	0.31	FW vs. DF	−0.05	[−0.7 to 0.6]	>0.999	−0.14 [−1.3 to 0.9]
	GK	M	3.20	FW vs. GK	0.13	[−0.6 to 0.9]	>0.999	0.34 [−0.9 to 1.7]
		SD	0.28	DF vs. GK	0.18	[−0.5 to 0.8]	>0.999	0.56 [−0.7 to 1.8]
COD (m.s)	HB	M	1.97	HB vs. WG	0.07	[−0.30 to 0.43]	>0.999	0.24 [−1.0 to 1.5]
		SD	0.21	HB vs. FW	0.15	[−0.19 to 0.49]	>0.999	0.75 [−0.5 to 1.9]
	WG	M	1.90	HB vs. DF	0.04	[−0.27 to 0.35]	>0.999	0.23 [−0.8 to 1.3]
		SD	0.30	HB vs. GK	0.01	[−0.36 to 0.37]	>0.999	0.04 [−1.2 to 1.3]
	FW	M	1.82	WG vs. FW	0.08	[−0.30 to 0.46]	>0.999	0.32 [−1.0 to 1.6]
		SD	0.14	WG vs. DF	−0.03	[−0.37 to 0.32]	>0.999	−0.13 [−1.3 to 1.1]
	DF	M	1.93	WG vs. GK	−0.06	[−0.46 to 0.34]	>0.999	−0.22 [−1.6 to 1.2]
		SD	0.12	FW vs. DF	−0.11	[−0.43 to 0.21]	>0.999	−0.81 [−1.9 to 0.4]
	GK	M	1.96	FW vs. GK	−0.14	[−0.52 to 0.24]	>0.999	−0.91 [−2.3 to 0.5]
		SD	0.14	DF vs. GK	−0.03	[−0.38 to 0.31]	>0.999	−0.24 [−1.5 to 0.9]
Peak Power (w)	HB	M	801.5	HB vs. WG	−55.3	[−232.0 to 121.5]	>0.999	−0.59 [−1.9 to 0.7]
		SD	103.3	HB vs. FW	206.3 *	[40.5 to 372.1]	0.008 #	1.83 [0.4 to 3.3]
	WG	M	856.8	HB vs. DF	−3.8	[−151.7 to 144.2]	>0.999	−0.03 [−1.1 to 1.0]
		SD	31.2	HB vs. GK	−86.3	[−263.0 to 90.5]	>0.999	−0.94 [−2.3 to 0.4]
	FW	M	595.2	WG vs. FW	261.5 *	[77.8 to 445.3]	0.002 #	2.91 [1.0 to 4.8]
		SD	102.0	WG vs. DF	51.5	[−116.2 to 219.2]	>0.999	0.55 [−0.7 to 1.8]
	DF	M	805.3	WG vs. GK	−31.0	[−224.7 to 162.7]	>0.999	−1.06 [−2.5 to 0.4]
		SD	100.6	FW vs. DF	−210.1 *	[−366.2 to −53.9]	0.004 #	−1.93 [−3.3 to −0.6]
	GK	M	887.8	FW vs. GK	−292.5 *	[−476.3 to −108.8]	0.001 #	−3.33 [−5.4 to −1.3]
		SD	17.7	DF vs. GK	−82.5	[−250.2 to 85.2]	>0.999	−0.90 [−2.2 to 0.6]
Fatigue index (%)	HB	M	41.3	HB vs. WG	−3.0	[−7.8 to 1.9]	0.685	−0.97 [−2.3 to 0.4]
		SD	2.3	HB vs. FW	−0.6	[−5.2 to 3.9]	>0.999	−0.24 [−1.4 to 0.9]
	WG	M	44.2	HB vs. DF	−2.1	[−6.2 to 1.9]	>0.999	−0.90 [−2.0 to 0.2]
		SD	3.5	HB vs. GK	−4.2	[−9.0 to 0.7]	0.134	−1.78 [−3.3 to −0.3]
	FW	M	41.9	WG vs. FW	2.4	[−2.7 to 7.4]	>0.999	0.73 [−0.6 to 2.1]
		SD	2.4	WG vs. DF	0.8	[−3.8 to 5.4]	>0.999	0.29 [−0.9 to 1.5]
	DF	M	43.4	WG vs. GK	−1.2	[−6.5 to 4.1]	>0.999	−0.38 [−1.8 to 1.0]
		SD	2.2	FW vs. DF	−1.5	[−5.8 to 2.8]	>0.999	−0.63 [−1.8 to 0.5]
	GK	M	45.4	FW vs. GK	−3.6	[−8.6 to 1.5]	0.379	−1.47 [−2.9 to 0.01]
		SD	1.8	DF vs. GK	−2.0	[−6.6 to 2.6]	>0.999	−0.91 [−2.2 to 0.4]

M, Mean; diff, difference; AcL, accumulated load training; COD = change of direction; VO_{2max}, maximal oxygen consumption; CM, central midfielder; WG, winger; FW, forward; DF, Defender; GK, goalkeeper; SD, standard deviation; A.U., arbitrary units; CI, confidence interval, and p, p-value at alpha level 0.05; Hedge's g (95% CI), Hedge's g effect size magnitude with 95% confidence interval. * The mean difference is significant at the 0.05 levels; # Indicates a significant difference.

Multiple linear regression analysis was calculated to predict the percentage of change in fitness levels (i.e., VO_{2max} (mL·kg^{-1}·min^{-1}) and peak power (PP, watts)) based on

AcL, BF%, maturity, somatotype, and baseline fitness levels in soccer player (Figure 2 and Table 4). The first analysis of VO_{2max} showed that there were significant ($F (8, 18) = 2.71$, $p = 0.038$), with a R^2 of just 0.55. Participants showed good predictions for VO_{2max}; (Y) is equal to Beta 0 + Beta1 (Acl) + Beta2 (BF%) + Beta3 (peak height velocity, PHV) + Beta4 (mesomorph) + Beta5 (sprint) + Beta6 (PP) + Beta7 (FI) + Beta8 (VO_{2max}), where AcL was measured as A.U, PHV was measured as years, fitness status was measured as COD (change of direction, seconds), PP (watts), FI (fatigue index, %), and VO_{2max} ($mL \cdot kg^{-1} \cdot min^{-1}$) in order based on the equation.

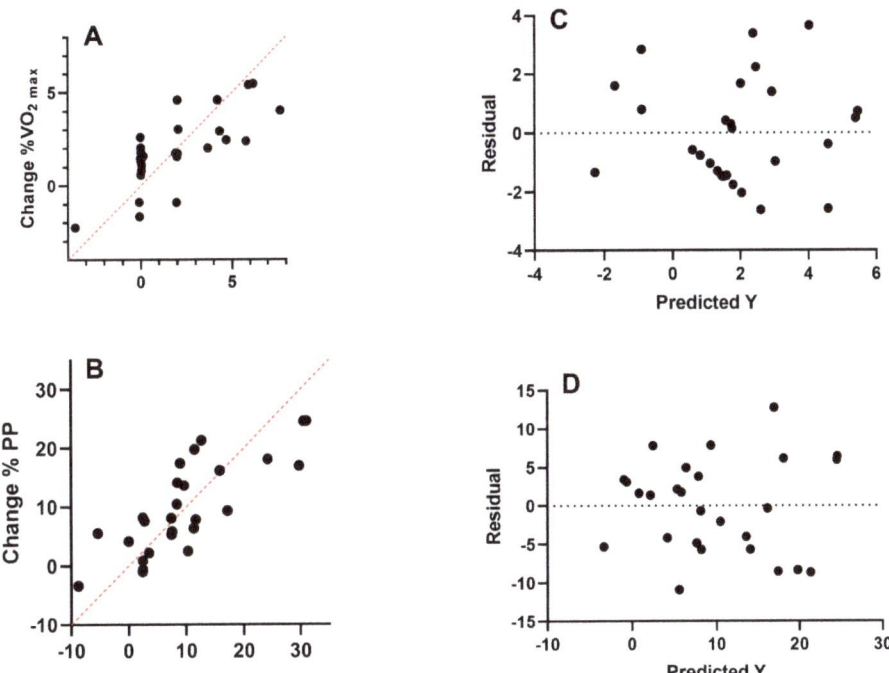

Figure 2. Multiple linear regression analysis was calculated to predict the percentage of change in fitness levels (**A**) VO_{2max} and (**B**) PP based on accumulated training load, body fat %, maturity, somatotype, and baseline fitness levels in the soccer players. Also, residual plot was calculated to predict the percentage of change in fitness levels (**C**) VO_{2max} and (**D**) PP; the difference between the actual value of the dependent variable and the value predicted by the residual provided. Note: VO_{2max} = maximal oxygen consumption ($mL \cdot kg^{-1} \cdot min^{-1}$); PP = Peak power (watts).

There was significant statically found in PP ($F (8, 18) = 3.80$, $p = 0.009$), with an R^2 of 0.63. Participants showed good predictions for PP; (Y) is equal to Beta 0 + Beta1 (Acl) + Beta2 (BF%) + Beta3 (maturity offset) + Beta4 (mesomorph) + Beta5 (COD) + Beta6 (PP) + Beta7 (FI) + Beta8 (VO_{2max}), where AcL was measured as A.U, maturity offset was measured as years, fitness status was measured as sprint (seconds), PP (watts), FI (%), and VO_{2max} ($mL \cdot kg^{-1} \cdot min^{-1}$) in order based on the equation.

Table 4. Multiple linear regression analysis: percentage of change in VO_{2max} and peak power with workload, body fat, maturity, somatotype, and baseline fitness levels.

Variables	Beta	Estimate	|t|	p Value	95% CI for Estimated	Total Predict
VO_{2max} (%)	β0	−42.79	2.11	0.049 *	−85.37 to −0.21	
AcL (A.U.)	β1	−0.0001	0.39	0.698	−0.0004 to 0.0003	
BF (%)	β2	0.31	1.92	0.070	−0.03 to 0.66	$R^2 = 0.55$
PHV (years)	β3	4.41	3.41	0.003 *	1.69 to 7.12	Adjusted $R^2 = 0.35$
Mesomorph	β4	0.30	0.49	0.628	−0.98 to 1.57	$p = 0.04$
COD (Seconds)	β5	1.76	0.62	0.542	−4.20 to 7.72	AIC = 126.28
Peak power (watts)	β6	−0.002	0.46	0.649	−0.01 to 0.01	
Fatigue index (%)	β7	−0.29	0.93	0.366	−0.98 to 0.38	
VO_{2max} (mL·kg^{-1}·min^{-1})	β8	−0.14	0.96	0.352	−0.45 to 0.17	
Variables	Beta	Estimate	|t|	p Value	95% CI for Estimated	Total Predict
Peak Power (%)	β0	−83.58	1.11	0.279	−241.2 to 74.04	
AcL (A.U.)	β1	0.001	1.05	0.308	−0.001 to 0.002	
BF (%)	β2	1.93	2.90	0.001 *	0.53 to 3.34	$R^2 = 0.63$
Maturity offset (yrs)	β3	6.11	0.92	0.372	−7.92 to 20.13	Adjusted $R^2 = 0.46$
Mesomorph	β4	−3.88	1.52	0.146	−9.24 to 1.48	$p = 0.01$
Sprint (Seconds)	β5	20.57	3.73	0.002 *	8.97 to 32.17	AIC = 193.12
Peak power (watts)	β6	−0.019	1.34	0.196	−0.05 to 0.011	
Fatigue index (%)	β7	−0.056	0.05	0.961	−2.42 to 2.31	
VO_{2max} (mL·kg^{-1}·min^{-1})	β8	0.10	0.19	0.844	−0.97 to 1.17	

Note: β0 = Y; CI = confidence interval; AIC = Akaike information criterion; AcL = accumulated load training; BF = body fat; PHV = Peak height velocity; COD = change of direction; VO_{2max} = maximal oxygen consumption; % = The the percentage of change in between assessments from pre to post-test; A.U. = arbitrary units; yrs = years. * The significant differences at the 0.05 levels.

4. Discussion

The purposes of this study were: (i) to describe anthropometric, maturation, and somatotype differences of players based on playing positions; (ii) to analyze variations of accumulated load training (AcL) and fitness parameters between playing positions; and (iii) to show a multiple linear regression analysis between the percentage of change in fitness levels and variables of AcL, body fat percentage (BF%), maturity, somatotype, and baseline fitness levels. In this context, the present study contributes to the existing literature, providing information about the variables mentioned in youth athletes of a professional soccer club.

Regarding the first aim of this study, it was found that goalkeepers (GK) presented higher height, weight, maturity offset, BF and lean body mass (LBM) than other positions. Then, the wingers (WG) showed significantly less BF than GK, and the others positions as well, but the central midfielders (CM) presented lower LBM than other positions. The results are similar to those found in under-16 Spanish soccer players [39] and under-17 Brazilian soccer players [40].

The somatotype results showed some differences between player positions. For instance, the CM and GK presented high endomorph values while WG, defenders (DF) and forwards (FW) presented high ectomorph values. These results are consistent with anthropometric and body composition variables from the present study. Also, it is possible to observe some differences by player positions when compared with the study of Fidelix et al. [40], where it was found that the morphological configuration of DF, FW and GK was classified as a balanced mesomorph, while midfield players were classified as ectomorph-mesomorphs; in the present study the morphological configuration of the majority of GK and FW was classified as endomorph ectomorph, while DF and WG were considered balanced ectomorph and CM as endomorph-ectomorph. Some years ago, Rienzi et al. [41] found that GK possessed different somatotype characteristics from the other field positions. Even before, Casajús and Aragonés [42] found higher endomorph values for GK. Gil et al. [39] observed that under-16 soccer players presented higher mesomorph values (2.3-4.3-3.1), but the present study presented more balanced data. Possible explanations for the present result could be associated with food habits from Iran and some genetic influence which was not controlled in the present study.

Despite some differences between player positions, there are some findings somewhat hard to explain. From the assessment in pre-season, it was shown that WG accumulated higher training loads than other positions and GK accumulated lower training loads than other positions. In agreement with these findings, there was a lower VO_{2max} for GK, while other positions presented similar values and WG the highest VO_{2max}. Also, higher fatigue index (FI) was shown for GK. However, sprint and change of direction (COD) was similar between positions, and peak power (PP) was higher for GK and WG, while FW presented the lowest value. Considering the anthropometric, somatotype, maturation and body composition assessment of the soccer players, the results are difficult to explain and it is not possible to identify a pattern for each player's position. Previously, it was suggested that players that accumulated higher training loads required higher levels of aerobic capacity [43]. This per se, is associated with higher fat-free mass [44]. On the one hand, in the scenario of the present study, GK presented higher LBM but lower VO_{2max}. On the other hand, GK presented higher BF which is in opposition to the statements of Goran et al. [44]. It is important to highlight that the results for VO_{2max} came from Yo-Yo intermittent recovery test level 1 (YYIRT1) and different results could occur with a continuous incremental and maximal test.

In the present study, the only players who showed characteristics different from other positions' somatotype were midfield players. The distance traveled by midfield players is significantly higher than that of backs and FW [45], suggesting that this playing position requires a higher level of aerobic capacity [35], which is strongly influenced by fat-free mass [45]. Also, GK presented lower training load accumulation and higher FI, but it is suggested that higher training load accumulation should lead to higher levels of fatigue [46]. In addition, it is suggested that players with a greater intermittent aerobic capacity have reduced fatigue [47] and vice-versa, which is supported by our study. Furthermore, we also speculate that the higher values for FI could be associated with the number of impacts with soil that GK suffered.

Previously, it was reported that the magnitude of the relationships between age, maturation, body dimensions and match running performance were position dependent. Within a single age-group in the present player sample, maturation had a substantial impact on match running performance, especially in attacking players. Coaches may need to consider players' maturity status when assessing their on-field playing performance [48]. The present study supports the mentioned findings; however, the GK presented the highest level of maturity offset and the FW the second highest level. Meanwhile, this study did not assess match running performance, but it measured AcL, which reflects internal training load perceived by the external load experienced. However, in this scenario, the GK presented the lowest values and the FW the second lowest values during pre-season, but after-season FW presented the highest values.

While Taylor [49] states that in soccer, the best players can reach VO_{2max} levels of 65–70 $mL·kg^{-1}·min^{-1}$, depending on their age, level of individual performance and position on the pitch, Slimani et al. [3] consider a wide range between 48 and 62 $mL·kg^{-1}·min^{-1}$ and specifically, by position, they reported 48.4–57.5 $mL·kg^{-1}·min^{-1}$ for GK, 53.2–62.8 $mL·kg^{-1}·min^{-1}$ for DF, 54.7–63 $mL·kg^{-1}·min^{-1}$ for CM, and 54.5–62.9 $mL·kg^{-1}·min^{-1}$ for FW. Regarding pre-season, our data seems to be in line for all FW, CM, WG and DF, which presented similar values between 48.6 and 50.1 $mL·kg^{-1}·min^{-1}$ with the exception of GK who presented the lowest value (41.5 $mL·kg^{-1}·min^{-1}$). In addition, it was shown that 55% of VO_{2max} variability and 63% of PP variability is explained by independent variables, respectively (see Table 4 and Figure 2). After-season, FW, CM, WG and DF revealed a slight increase with a range between 49.6 and 51.6 $mL·kg^{-1}·min^{-1}$, with GK presenting 41.9 $mL·kg^{-1}·min^{-1}$.

In the present study of twenty-seven under-16 elite soccer players from the Iranian League, what have been found are significant relationships between VO_{2max} and peak height velocity (PHV) and between peak power with BF and peak power with sprint (all, $p < 0.05$, Table 4);recently [28], it was suggested that the higher physical capacity allows soccer players to perform with stronger exertion, which could be expressed in the values of the chronic workload and the accumulated training monotony. The same study found a relationship between the PHV and the accumulated training monotony, and between chronic workload and physical abilities that can be expressed by VO_{2max} [28].

Due to the limited sample of our study, we suggest larger samples with the same analysis to better interpret if the other variables, such as, AcL, maturity, somatotype and baseline fitness levels can predict VO_{2max} and peak power.

Higher VO_{2max} is associated with higher performance in matches such as distance traveled, intensity, number of sprints, and the amount of player involvement with the ball [50]. Also, soccer players will have more energy to move with few limitations and will have a fast recovery without increasing fatigue substantially. The statements presented regarding VO_{2max} supported some results found in the present study during pre-season. For instance, in pre-season, the position with higher VO_{2max} was WG, which was also revealed to be the position with higher AcL and more sprints. However, they did not present higher values of PP and COD tests. Possible explanations for these differences could be associated with the use of non-specific tests to assess PP for soccer players by using a bicycle ergometer; COD testing is a skill that could be developed with special care considering a specific position. After-season, the position with higher VO_{2max} was CM, but this time it only displays higher results in COD tests while other tests analyzed present different player positions with higher values (see Table 3). Despite the possible physiological and positional adaptations that may occur during the season, a justification for the presented results could be associated with previous studies that stated that in-season training load variability is very limited, and that only minor decrements or a maintenance during the season might occur [51–54], which is in line with Malone et al. [13], who posit that it is the need to win matches that influences a possible specific peak for strength and conditioning.

In agreement with Fidelix et al. [40] study, there are some limitations regarding our participants, as they belong to the same team which per se can be associated with a specific somatotype profile of the club's intention, its geographical location and others. Also, the small sample size and their specific team and country do not allow generalizing the present finding.

This study provides useful information regarding the AcL, anthropometric, body composition, maturity, somatotype and fitness levels such as VO_{2max}, PP, anaerobic power, aerobic power, COD, sprint and YYIRT1 of a youth soccer team during different in-season periods. It provides further evidence of the value of using a combination of different monitoring and assessment measures to fully evaluate the youth soccer player across a full competitive season. Moreover, it identifies differences between player positions which allow coaches, staff, and the scientific community to analyze youth soccer player with greater knowledge. Also, for coaches, this study could provide important information to be considered when planning training sessions and/or weekly periodization. For instance, coaches can use information from RPE to produce AcL and to better understand the load perceived by young soccer players. In addition, with the information from the present study, it is suggested to include the following fitness parameters when analyzing young soccer players: PHV, body composition variables such BF, somatotype, VO_{2max}, sprint and COD tests.

In future studies, it would be interesting to replicate the present study with more teams in the same season, level of competition, or even with different age groups to better interpretation of the results. Furthermore, it would be pertinent to replicate the present study with female soccer players and different age categories in order to increase knowledge on the variables analyzed.

5. Conclusions

In general, GK showed higher values in anthropometric, body composition variables and maturity offset compared to the other positions. In the opposite direction, WG presented lower levels of BF. In addition, there was only one significant difference in somatotype, where DF presented a higher endomorph value than WG.

Furthermore, there were several differences in the beginning of the season and few after-season. In pre-season, AcL, VO_{2max}, sprint was found to be higher for WG while COD was found to be higher for CM. PP and FI was found to be higher for GK. After-season, AcL, is similar for all positions except for the GK. VO_{2max} was found to be higher for CM. Sprint was higher for WG. COD was found to be higher for CM and GK. Still, PP and FI was found to be higher for GK. These finding reinforce the tactical role of the positions as they produce different adaptations during the season. Our multiple linear regressions support these findings because they indicated that our model explains more than 50% of all the variability of the responses.

This information is useful for coaches and professionals involved in sports, as it can be used in the process of talent selection and the development of training programs because they serve as a reference for athletes of the same sex, age and competitive level.

Author Contributions: Conceptualization, H.N., R.O., J.P.-G. and L.P.A.; methodology, H.N., R.O., F.M.C., E.P.-M. and J.P.-G.; software, H.N., F.M.C., R.O. and J.P.-G.; formal analysis, H.N., F.M.C., and R.O.; investigation, J.P.-G., H.N. and R.O.; writing—original draft preparation, H.N. and R.O.; writing—review and editing, H.N., E.P.-M., R.O., J.P.-G. and L.P.A. All authors have read and agreed to the published version of the manuscript.

Funding: Portuguese Foundation for Science and Technology, I.P., Grant/Award Number UIDP/04748/2020.

Institutional Review Board Statement: The study was conducted according to the guidelines of the Declaration of Helsinki, and approved by the Ethics Committee of the Ethics Committee of the Sport Sciences Research Institute (IR.SSRC.REC.1399.060).

Informed Consent Statement: Informed consent was obtained from all subjects and their parents involved in the study.

Data Availability Statement: The datasets used and/or analyzed during the current study are available from the corresponding author on reasonable request.

Acknowledgments: The authors would like to thank the team's coaches and players for their cooperation during all data collection procedures.

Conflicts of Interest: The authors declare no conflict of interest.

References

1. Nikolaidis, P.T.; Ziv, G.; Lidor, R.; Arnon, M. Intra-individual variability in soccer players of different age groups playing different positions. *J. Hum. Kinet.* **2014**, *40*, 1–13. [CrossRef]
2. Castillo, D.; Los Arcos, A.; Martinez-Santos, R. Aerobic endurance performance does not determine the professional career of elite youth soccer players. *J. Sports Med. Phys. Fit.* **2018**, *58*, 392–398. [CrossRef]
3. Nobari, H.; Vahabi, R.; Pérez-Gómez, J.; Ardigò, L.P. Variations of Training Workload in Micro-and Meso-cycles Based on Position in Elite Young Soccer Players: One season study. *Front. Physiol.* **2021**, *12*, 529. [CrossRef]
4. Slimani, M.; Znazen, H.; Miarka, B.; Bragazzi, N.L. Maximum Oxygen Uptake of Male Soccer Players According to their Competitive Level, Playing Position and Age Group: Implication from a Network Meta-Analysis. *J. Hum. Kinet.* **2019**, *66*, 233–245. [CrossRef]
5. Mujika, I.; Vaeyens, R.; Matthys, S.P.J.; Santisteban, J.; Goiriena, J.; Philippaerts, R. The relative age effect in a professional football club setting. *J. Sports Sci.* **2009**, *27*, 1153–1158. [CrossRef] [PubMed]
6. Carter, J.E.L.; Heath, B.H. *Somatotyping: Development and Applications*; Cambridge University Press: Cambridge, UK, 1990.
7. Eston, R.; Reilly, T. *Kinanthropometry and Exercise Physiology Laboratory Manual: Tests, Procedures and Data: Volume Two: Physiology*; Routledge: London, UK, 2013; pp. 23–30.
8. Chamari, K.; Hachana, Y.; Ahmed, Y.B.; Galy, O.; Sghaier, F.; Chatard, J.C.; Hue, O.; Wisloff, U. Field and laboratory testing in young elite soccer players. *Br. J. Sports Med.* **2004**, *38*, 191–196. [CrossRef]

9. Moghadam, M.M.; Azarbayjani, M.A.; Sadeghi, H. The comparison of the anthropometric characteristics of Iranian elite male soccer players in different game position. *J. Sport Sci.* **2012**, *6*, 393–400.
10. Nobari, H.; Silva, A.F.; Clemente, F.M.; Siahkouhian, M.; García-Gordillo, M.A.; Adsuar, J.C.; Pérez-Gómez, J. Analysis of Fitness Status Variations of Under-16 Soccer Players Over a Season and Their Relationships With Maturational Status and Training Load. *Front. Physiol.* **2021**, *11*, 1840. [CrossRef] [PubMed]
11. Di Salvo, V.; Baron, R.; Tschan, H.; Calderon Montero, F.J.; Bachi, N.; Pigozzi, F. Performance characteristics according to playing position in elite soccer. *Int. J. Sports Med.* **2007**, *28*, 222–227. [CrossRef]
12. Nobari, H.; Alves, A.R.; Clemente, F.M.; Pérez-Gómez, J.; Clark, C.C.T.; Granacher, U.; Zouhal, H. Associations Between Variations in Accumulated Workload and Physiological Variables in Young Male Soccer Players Over the Course of a Season. *Front. Physiol.* **2021**, *12*, 233. [CrossRef] [PubMed]
13. Nobari, H.; Kargarfard, M.; Minasian, V.; Cholewa, J.M.; Pérez-Gómez, J. The effects of 14-week betaine supplementation on endocrine markers, body composition and anthropometrics in professional youth soccer players: A double blind, randomized, placebo-controlled trial. *J. Int. Soc. Sports Nutr.* **2021**, *18*, 20. [CrossRef]
14. Bahtra, R.; Asmawi, M.; Dlis, F. Improved VO2Max: The Effectiveness of Basic Soccer Training at a Young Age. *Int. J. Hum. Mov. Sports Sci.* **2020**, *8*, 97–102. [CrossRef]
15. Markovic, G.; Mikulic, P. Discriminative ability of the yo-yo intermittent recovery test (level 1) in prospective young soccer players. *J. Strength Cond. Res.* **2011**, *25*, 2931–2934. [CrossRef]
16. Jones, C.M.; Griffiths, P.C.; Mellalieu, S.D. Training load and fatigue marker associations with injury and illness: A systematic review of longitudinal studies. *Sports Med.* **2017**, *47*, 943–974. [CrossRef] [PubMed]
17. Nobari, H.; Fani, M.; Clemente, F.M.; Carlos-Vivas, J.; Pérez-Gómez, J.; Ardigò, L.P. Intra- and Inter-week Variations of Well-Being Across a Season: A Cohort Study in Elite Youth Male Soccer Players. *Front. Physiol.* **2021**, *12*, 1030. [CrossRef]
18. Malone, J.; Di Michele, R.; Morgans, R.; Burgess, D.; Morton, J.; Drust, B. Seasonal Training-Load Quantification in Elite English Premier League Soccer Players. *Int. J. Sports Physiol. Perform.* **2015**, *10*, 489–497. [CrossRef] [PubMed]
19. Nobari, H.; Akyildiz, Z.; Fani, M.; Oliveira, R.; Pérez-Gómez, J.; Clemente, F.M. Weekly Wellness Variations to Identify Non-Functional Overreaching Syndrome in Turkish National Youth Wrestlers: A Pilot Study. *Sustainability* **2021**, *13*, 4667. [CrossRef]
20. Haddad, M.; Stylianides, G.; Djaoui, L.; Dellal, A.; Chamari, K. Session-RPE Method for Training Load Monitoring: Validity, Ecological Usefulness, and Influencing Factors. *Front. Neurol.* **2017**, *11*. [CrossRef] [PubMed]
21. Nobari, H.; Barjaste, A.; Haghighi, H.; Clemente, F.M.; Carlos-Vivas, J.; Perez-Gomez, J. Quantification of training and match load in elite youth soccer players: A full-season study. *J. Sports Med. Phys. Fit.* **2021**. [CrossRef]
22. American College of Sports Medicine. *ACSM's Guidelines for Exercise Testing and Prescription*; Lippincott Williams & Wilkins: Philadelphia, PA, USA, 2014.
23. Jackson, A.S.; Pollock, M.L. Generalized equations for predicting body density of men. *Br. J. Nutr.* **1978**, *40*, 497–504. [CrossRef] [PubMed]
24. Nobari, H.; Aquino, R.; Clemente, F.M.; Khalafi, M.; Adsuar, J.C.; Pérez-Gómez, J. Description of acute and chronic load, training monotony and strain over a season and its relationships with well-being status: A study in elite under-16 soccer players. *Physiol. Behav.* **2020**, *225*, 113117. [CrossRef] [PubMed]
25. Arazi, H.; Mirzaei, B.; Nobari, H. Anthropometric profile, body composition and somatotyping of national Iranian cross-country runners. *Turk J. Sport Exerc.* **2015**, *17*, 35–41. [CrossRef]
26. Rahmat, A.J.; Arsalan, D.; Bahman, M.; Hadi, N. Anthropometrical profile and bio-motor abilities of young elite wrestlers. *Phys. Educ. Stud.* **2016**, *6*, 63–69. [CrossRef]
27. Sheppard, J.M.; Young, W.B. Agility literature review: Classifications, training and testing. *J. Sports Sci.* **2006**, *24*, 919–932. [CrossRef]
28. Nobari, H.; Tubagi Polito, L.F.; Clemente, F.M.; Pérez-Gómez, J.; Ahmadi, M.; Garcia-Gordillo, M.Á.; Silva, A.F.; Adsuar, J.C. Relationships between training workload parameters with variations in anaerobic power and change of direction status in elite youth soccer players. *Int. J. Environ. Res. Public Health* **2020**, *17*, 7934. [CrossRef]
29. Mirkov, D.; Nedeljkovic, A.; Kukolj, M.; Ugarkovic, D.; Jaric, S. Evaluation of the reliability of soccer-specific field tests. *J. Strength Cond. Res.* **2008**, *22*, 1046–1050. [CrossRef]
30. Vandewalle, D.; Gilbert, P.; Monod, H. Standard anaerobic tests. *Sports Med.* **1987**, *4*, 268–289. [CrossRef] [PubMed]
31. Bar-Or, O. The Wingate anaerobic test: An update on methodology, reliability and validity. *Sports Med.* **1987**, *4*, 381–394. [CrossRef]
32. Bangsbo, J.; Iaia, F.M.; Krustrup, P. The Yo-Yo intermittent recovery test. *Sports Med.* **2008**, *38*, 37–51. [CrossRef]
33. Borg, G. Perceived exertion as an indicator of somatic stress. *Scand. J. Rehab. Med.* **1970**, *2*, 92–98.
34. Nobari, H.; Silva, R.; Clemente, F.M.; Akyildiz, Z.; Ardigò, L.P.; Pérez-Gómez, J. Weekly Variations in the Workload of Turkish National Youth Wrestlers: A Season of Complete Preparation. *Int. J. Environ. Res. Public Health* **2021**, *18*, 3832. [CrossRef]
35. Foster, C.A. Monitoring training in athletes with reference to overtraining syndrome. *Occup. Health Ind. Med.* **1998**, *4*, 189. [CrossRef] [PubMed]
36. Foster, C.; Florhaug, J.A.; Franklin, J.; Gottschall, L.; Hrovatin, L.A.; Parker, S.; Doleshal, P.; Dodge, C. A new approach to monitoring exercise training. *J. Strength Cond. Res.* **2001**, *15*, 109–115.

37. Hopkins, W.; Marshall, S.; Batterham, A.; Hanin, J. Progressive statistics for studies in sports medicine and exercise science. *Med. Sci. Sports Exerc.* **2009**, *41*, 3. [CrossRef]
38. Baumgartner, T.A.; Chung, H. Confidence Limits for Intraclass Reliability Coefficients. *Meas. Phys. Educ. Exerc. Sci.* **2001**, *5*, 179–188. [CrossRef]
39. Gil, S.M.; Gil, J.; Ruiz, F.; Irazusta, A.; Irazusta, J. Anthropometrical characteristics and somatotype of young soccer players and their comparison with the general population. *Biol. Sport* **2010**, *27*, 17–24. [CrossRef]
40. Fidelix, Y.L.; Berria, J.; Ferrari, E.P.; Ortiz, J.G.; Cetolin, T.; Petroski, E.L. Somatotype of Competitive Youth Soccer Players from Brazil. *J. Hum. Kinet.* **2014**, *42*, 259–266. [CrossRef] [PubMed]
41. Rienzi, E.; Drust, B.; Reilly, T.; Carter, J.E.; Martin, A. Investigation of anthropometric and work-rate profiles of elite South American international soccer players. *J. Sports Med. Phys. Fit.* **2000**, *40*, 162–169.
42. Casajús, J.; Aragonés, M.T. Morphological study of high-level soccer players. Body composition and Somatotype. *Arch. Med. Deporte* **1991**, *8*, 147–151.
43. Reilly, T. Energetics of high-intensity exercise (soccer) with particular reference to fatigue. *J. Sport Sci.* **1997**, *15*, 257–263. [CrossRef] [PubMed]
44. Goran, M.; Fields, D.A.; Hunter, G.R.; Herd, S.L.; Weinsier, R.L. Total body fat does not influence maximal aerobic capacity. *Int. J. Obes. Relat. Metab. Disord.* **2000**, *24*, 841–848. [CrossRef] [PubMed]
45. Reilly, T.; Bangsbo, J.; Franks, A. Anthropometric and physiological predispositions for elite soccer. *J. Sport Sci.* **2000**, *18*, 669–683. [CrossRef] [PubMed]
46. Lovell, R.; Fransen, J.; Ryan, R.; Massard, T.; Cross, R.; Eggers, T.; Duffield, R. Biological maturation and match running performance: A national football (soccer) federation perspective. *J. Sci. Med. Sport* **2019**. [CrossRef] [PubMed]
47. Rampinini, E.; Impellizzeri, F.M.; Castagna, C.; Azzalin, A.; Bravo, D.F.; Wisløff, U. Effect of match-related fatigue on short-passing ability in young soccer players. *Med. Sci. Sports Exerc.* **2008**, *40*, 934–942. [CrossRef]
48. Buchheit, M.; Mendez-Villanueva, A. Effects of age, maturity and body dimensions on match running performance in highly trained under-15 soccer players. *J. Sports Sci.* **2014**, *32*, 1271–1278. [CrossRef] [PubMed]
49. Taylor, J. Youth Football. Available online: https://resources.fifa.com/image/upload/youth-football-training-manual-2866317.pdf?cloudid=mxpozhvr2gjshmxrilpf.
50. Russell, M.; Sparkes, W.; Northeast, J.; Cook, C.J.; Love, T.D.; Bracken, R.M.; Kilduff, L. Changes in acceleration and deceleration capacity throughout professional soccer match-play. *J. Strength Cond. Res.* **2016**, *30*, 2839–2844. [CrossRef]
51. Nobari, H.; Oliveira, R.; Clemente, F.M.; Adsuar, J.C.; Pérez-Gómez, J.; Carlos-Vivas, J.; Brito, J.P. Comparisons of Accelerometer Variables Training Monotony and Strain of Starters and Non-Starters: A Full-Season Study in Professional Soccer Players. *Int. J. Environ. Res. Public Health* **2020**, *17*, 6547. [CrossRef]
52. Oliveira, R.; Brito, J.P.; Loureiro, N.; Padinha, V.; Ferreira, B.; Mendes, B. Does the distribution of the weekly training load account for the match results of elite professional soccer players? *Physiol. Behav.* **2020**, *225*, 113118. [CrossRef]
53. Oliveira, R.; Brito, J.P.; Martins, A.; Mendes, B.; Calvete, F.; Carriço, S.; Ferraz, R.; Marques, M. In-season training load quantification of one-, two- and three-game week schedules in a top European professional soccer team. *Physiol. Behav.* **2019**, *201*, 146–156. [CrossRef] [PubMed]
54. Oliveira, R.; Brito, J.P.; Martins, A.; Mendes, B.; Ferraz, R.; Marques, M. In-season internal and external training load quantification of an elite European soccer team. *PLoS ONE* **2019**, *14*, e0209393. [CrossRef]

MDPI
St. Alban-Anlage 66
4052 Basel
Switzerland
Tel. +41 61 683 77 34
Fax +41 61 302 89 18
www.mdpi.com

Children Editorial Office
E-mail: children@mdpi.com
www.mdpi.com/journal/children

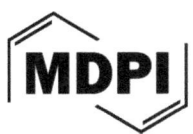

www.ingramcontent.com/pod-product-compliance
Lightning Source LLC
LaVergne TN
LVHW070547100526
838202LV00012B/404